Burns and their treatment

Burns and their treatment

Third Edition

I. F. K. Muir, MBE, VRD, MB, MS, FRCS, FRCS(Ed)

Clinical Senior Lecturer in Surgery, University of Aberdeen; formerly Consultant in Plastic Surgery, Aberdeen General and Special Hospitals

T. L. Barclay, MB, ChM, FRCS, FRCS(Ed)

Formerly Consultant Plastic Surgeon, Bradford Royal Infirmary and St Luke's Hospital, Bradford; formerly Consultant Surgeon in Charge, Yorkshire Regional Burns Centre, Pinderfields Hospital, Wakefield

and

John A. D. Settle, OBE, MPhil, MRCS, LRCP, DA

Consultant in Clinical Physiology; Director, Yorkshire Regional BurnsCentre, Pinderfields General Hospital, Wakefield; Honorary Clinical Lecturer, Department of Surgery, University of Leeds

Butterworths

London   Boston   Durban   Singapore   Sydney   Toronto   Wellington

First published by Lloyd-Luke (Medical Books) Ltd, 1962
Second edition, 1974
Third edition published by Butterworths, 1987

© **Butterworth & Co. (Publishers) Ltd, 1987**

British Library Cataloguing in Publication Data

Muir, I. F. K.
   Burns and their treatment.—3rd ed.
   1. Burns and scalds
   I. Title   II. Barclay, T. L.   III. Settle, John, A. D.
   617'.1106   RD96.4

   ISBN 0-407-00333-9

Library of Congress Cataloging-in-Publication Data

Muir, Ian F. K. (Ian Fraser Kerr)
   Burns and their treatment.

   Includes bibliographies and index.
   1. Burns and scalds. I. Barclay, T. L. (Thomas Laird)
2. Settle, John A. D. III. Title.
[DNLM: 1. Burns—therapy. W0 704 M953b]
RD96.4.M83   1987   617'.11   86-31060

   ISBN 0-407-00333-9

Photoset by Butterworths Litho Preparation Department
Printed and bound in Great Britain by Butler & Tanner, Frome, Somerset

Foreword to the first edition

Almost invariably burns are incurred through carelessness and are paid as the price of civilization. It is unfortunate that children and the elderly should bear the brunt of our apparent unwillingness to screen our fires, to protect our cookers and to elaborate methods of rendering clothing less inflammable. Whatever the causes more than 14 000 sufferers are treated in hospital every year, but this figure represents only one-tenth of the problem, since the numbers dealt with by general practitioners or by 'self help' remain a matter of conjecture.

The more extensive injuries present an immediate threat to life. Subsequent treatment will be prolonged and may well fail to result in the restoration of anything like full function. All but the most minor lesions will cause disfiguring scars which must to a large extent be permanent.

From time immemorial there have been a multiplicity of treatments suggested for burns and it is suggested that this can be regarded as an index of our ignorance of the subject. On the other hand it could be an admission of the vast differences existing between one burn and another and between their effects, both immediate and remote, on different individuals. Area, depth and site are important, whilst the age of the sufferer may well be a determining factor.

It will be evident that much knowledge has been acquired and it may be that our greatest lack is not of knowledge, but of the clinical skill and the amenities requisite to ensure its correct and timely application.

The book reflects the experiences of experts working in a centre specially adapted and equipped to deal first with the illness created by burns, then with the recreation of an intact skin surface and finally, wherever this is possible, with the restoration of lost function. As the result of such work here and elsewhere, recovery can be expected to be more rapid and more complete and to be achieved at the expense of less pain and suffering than hitherto. There has, however, been but little if any alteration in mortality rates.

There is no question but that the treatment of all phases of an extensive burn injury taxes the skill and the knowledge of the surgeon to the utmost. The difference between success and failure may depend as much on an evaluation of the individual patient as it does on technical procedures. In essence this is true of all reparative medicine and surgery – care expended on the evaluation of these factors influences both immediate survival and ultimate function. The writers are not afraid to point out that there can be occasions when enthusiastic resuscitation may well not result in the remote possibility of recovery, but only in the prolongation of the agony of dying.

It is certain that anyone from the most recent graduate to the most senior consultant will find in these pages explicit guidance without didacticism. He will be left with a clear appreciation both of the enormity of the problem posed by any extensive burn and of the means presently at our disposal to ensure that the end result in functional and cosmetic restoration is as nearly perfect as may be and that such a state shall be achieved in the least possible time and with minimal suffering.

Rainsford Mowlem
July 1962

Preface to the third edition

Since the date of the second edition eleven years ago, there have been no fundamental changes in our approach to the problems of burns. There have, however, been a number of technical developments which have given improved results.

In the United Kingdom, the number and severity of burns remain a serious problem but legislation and changed social habits, particularly in the field of clothing, in the heating of homes, and in other domestic factors, have resulted in a change in the incidence of different types of injury.

The use of colloids in the treatment of shock has decreased and in many countries treatment is entirely or predominantly by electrolytes.

The basic techniques for the prevention and treatment of infection are unchanged but new antiseptics and antibiotics are additional weapons in the therapeutic armoury.

These new reagents and other factors which have improved the general condition of patients have enabled surgeons to give more attention to improving the quality of healing, the operation of tangential excision and overgrafting being one of the important techniques which has been developed from this end.

John Settle has joined the two original authors for this third edition.

IFKM, TLB and JADS

Preface to the first edition

In *A System of Surgery* by Holmes and Walker published in 1883 are to be found the following words:

'The local treatment of burns is a subject on which many books have been written and perhaps more numerous remedies recommended than in any branch of surgery. The success which is said to have attended very different, and even opposite modes of treatment, shows that the authors must either be misrepresenting the facts or speaking about different matters. I prefer the latter explanation, more especially as I find authors who have written to recommend certain methods have almost invariably spoken of burns as if they were all alike, forgetful, apparently, that the essential question in the treatment of a burn is the depth or degree, the consequent probability of sloughing, ulceration, or mere inflammation resembling erysipelas. It is only by keeping this point steadily in view that we can hope to arrive at any rational plan for the treatment of these injuries.'

These words remain a pertinent comment on the treatment of burns at the present day. Since they were written, the treatment of burns has changed in many ways, and publications on the subject have appeared and continue to appear with great frequency. The very number and variety of recommendations for treatment make it clear that there is still no single 'best treatment' for burns, and in order to make the best use of modern materials and techniques, the doctor must be able to choose the method of treatment which is most suitable for the individual patient under the particular circumstances of the moment.

Registrars, casualty officers and house surgeons are most likely to have the responsibility of initiating treatment and supervising the day-to-day care of patients, yet they are unlikely to have had sufficient experience to be able to evaluate the many and apparently contradictory recommendations.

In this book we have attempted to go into the rationale behind various methods of treatment and to give the reasons for our own choice of methods. We make no apology for discussing certain simple but important subjects at some length, for, as in other branches of medicine and surgery, it is only by a constant awareness of the basic principles involved that intelligent use can be made of the methods available.

A mass of information from the laboratory workers' standpoint has been collected and analysed by Sevitt in his book *Burns – Pathology and Therapeutic Applications* (Butterworth, 1957); and Artz and Reiss in *The Treatment of Burns* (W. B. Saunders, 1957) have given an account of clinical practice in the USA. The present book is based on current practice in Great Britain, and more particularly on that in the wards of the Mount Vernon Centre for Plastic Surgery.

Both of us have been fortunate enough to serve as senior registrars under Mr Rainsford Mowlem, surgeon-in-charge of the Mount Vernon Centre for Plastic Surgery, and we are fully conscious of the debt which we owe to him for our understanding of the problems of the care of burned patients. We hope that we have been able to pass on some of the clarity of his thought and teaching. We are also grateful to our colleagues at Mount Vernon, R. L. G. Dawson and S. H. Harrison for their cooperation and help.

It is a pleasure also to acknowledge our indebtedness to workers in other units, and in particular to D. McG. Jackson and his colleagues of Birmingham, A. B. Wallace and A. D. R. Batchelor of Edinburgh, T. Gibson of Glasgow and A. J. Evans of Roehampton.

The photographic illustrations are the work of the photographers at our various hospitals and we acknowledge our gratitude for their help; Miss Susan Robinson kindly prepared the line diagrams.

We are grateful to Parke-Davis and Co. of Hounslow, and Smith and Nephew of Welwyn Garden City who have made generous contributions towards the cost of the coloured illustrations.

IFKM and TLB

Contents

Chapter 1

The scope of the burns problem

During the last 20 years, deaths from burns and scalds in England and Wales have declined by 12 per cent in actual numbers and by 20 per cent when calculated as deaths per million of population. In spite of this welcome improvement, there are still over 600 deaths each year and more than 10 000 people who require hospital treatment, surviving with varying degrees of disfigurement and disability.

Patients with burns and scalds fall into distinct age categories: under the age of 3 scalds predominate, from ages 3 to 14 most injuries are due to clothes catching fire or are the result of conflagration, from age 15 to 60 industrial accidents predominate, whilst after the age of 60 the general effects of ageing result in an increased risk of thermal injury. In almost all age groups, there are proportionally more burn injuries to males than to females. It is instructive to consider the incidence in some detail because this indicates the variety of injuries and the types of patients likely to present at the accident department. Furthermore, it illustrates the effectiveness of previous preventive measures and identifies where further effort is most required.

Incidence

The exact incidence of patients with burns and scalds in England and Wales who require admission to hospital is not known, but a reliable estimate can be derived from data published by the Department of Health and Social Security (1981) in the form of the *Hospital In-Patient Enquiry*. This is based on a 10 per cent sample of all discharges and deaths from National Health Service hospitals in England and Wales to which a factor of 10 is then applied. These data for 1981, presented as burns per 10 000 population in each of seven age groups, are shown as a histogram in *Figure 1.1*. The most striking features are that the risk factor for children under five is eight times greater than for the rest of the population and that people over 75 years of age are twice as likely to be burned or scalded than are the rest of the adult population.

By the use of the 1981 population census figures on which these rates of incidence are based, it is possible to derive the estimated number of patients with burns and scalds treated as in-patients in England and Wales during 1981. This produces a total of 10 960 patients made up almost equally of 5510 children (0–14 years) and 5450 adults. The numbers in each of the seven age groups are shown as a histogram in *Figure 1.2*. These data reveal that, after young children, the next largest group of

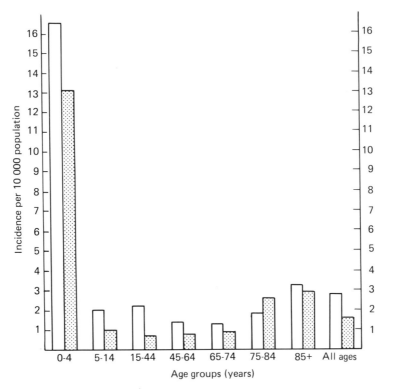

Figure 1.1 Incidence of patients with burns or scalds admitted to hospital in England and Wales during 1981.   □ Males;   ▦ females

burn patients requiring admission to hospital consists of young adult males (15–44 years) who comprise 21 per cent of the total. It is also interesting to note that although elderly patients (75+ years) account for only 6.5 per cent of the total, three-quarters of these patients are female, whilst in all other age groups males predominate.

The pattern of admission to specialized burn centres is similar but shows a slight preponderance of adults. This probably results from a high proportion of young children with small scalds whose treatment is adequately provided for in paediatric wards. The admission figures for the North-West Regional Burns Centre, Mount Vernon Hospital, Northwood in the period 1954–59, and the Yorkshire Regional Burns Centre, Pinderfields Hospital, Wakefield in the years 1966–83 are shown below together with the England and Wales total for 1981.

	Mount Vernon *1954–59* *(862 patients)*	*Pinderfields* *1966–83* *(1429 patients)*	*England and Wales* *1981* *(10 960 patients)*
Children 0–14	46.3%	45.8%	50.3%
Adult 15–64	46.5%	43.3%	38.7%
Adult 65+	7.2%	10.9%	11.0%
Children:Adults	1:1.16	1:1.18	1:0.99

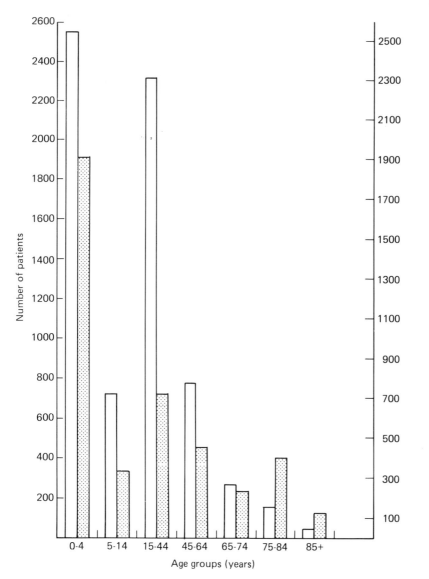

Figure 1.2 Actual numbers of patients with burns or scalds admitted to hospital in England and Wales during 1981. ☐ Males; ▦ females

Children

The pattern of injury in children differs markedly in different age groups and correlates with the different interests and abilities of the child as development occurs. Children of less than 9 months are not mobile and most thermal injuries to these infants result from hot liquids being spilled onto them. However, towards the end of its first year, the active child can easily pull the arm of an adult holding a hot drink or pull the cord of an electric kettle on a nearby work-top. Between 1 and 5 years the child is increasingly mobile, inquisitive, touches everything within reach, but does not yet understand many of the hazards of everyday life. Up to the age of 5 years, more than three-quarters of the thermal injuries are scalds and three-quarters of these are caused by spillage from cups, pots, kettles and pans as the child reaches for containers of hot liquids or pulls tableclothes, kettle cords or pan handles. The older child has learned about most of these hazards but has accidents in the handling of kettles and pans and is more likely to suffer the very serious accident of falling into a bath of hot water.

The causes of thermal injury in children and their relative importance in different age groups are shown in *Figure 1.3* using data from the Department of Trade (1983) study of domestic thermal injury. Of the 665 thermal injuries studied, 72 per cent were in children under the age of 5; of these 477 injuries, 78 per cent were scalds. The declining incidence of scalds and the inverse rising incidence of flame burns with increasing age is very obvious. Contact burns occurred only in children under

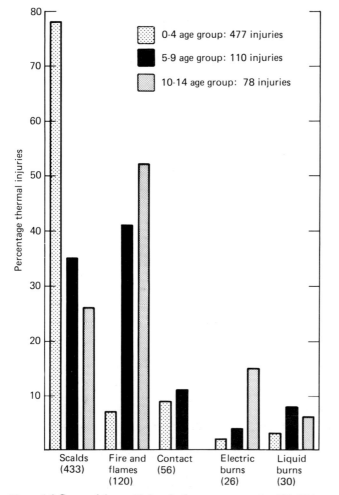

Figure 1.3 Cause of thermal injury in three age groups for 665 children

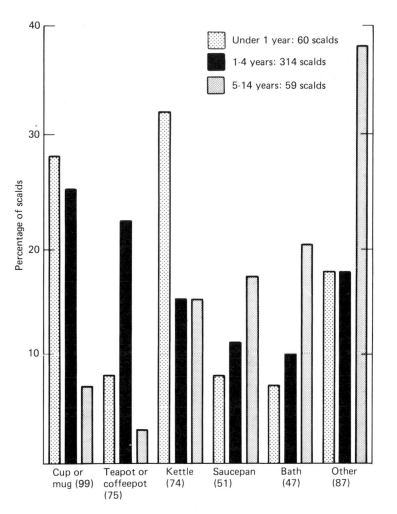

Figure 1.4 Cause of scalds in three age groups for 433 children

10 in this series, whilst electrical current burns were a significant cause of injury in the 10–14 age group.

Analysis of the 433 scalds to show the relative importance of different mechanisms in different age groups is shown in *Figure 1.4*. In the under 1 year age group, cups and kettles accounted for 60 per cent of the scalds, but only 22 per cent of those in the 5–14 year group. The increasing importance of pans and baths as causes of scalds in older children is clearly shown. Analysis of the source of ignition for the 120 fire and flame burns revealed that small sources, such as matches, cigarettes and candles, were responsible for 34 per cent of the injuries. Outdoor bonfires and barbecues etc. accounted for 22 per cent, space heating (domestic fires) for 11 per cent, cooking equipment for 10 per cent and house fires for 7 per cent. In 60 per cent of the 120 cases clothing caught fire and in 30 per cent a flammable liquid was involved in some way.

The third largest group of children in the study of the Department of Trade (1983) shown in *Figure 1.3* are those who were injured by contact with a hot object. These typically are injuries of very young children; 44 of the 56 were under 5 years of age and 34 were under 2 years of age. Although the commonest single cause was contact with an iron (11 cases), the second commonest – contact with an electric bar fire (9 cases) – is by far the most serious since it can produce full thickness destruction to much of the skin of the palm and palmar surface of the fingers.

Adults of working age (15–64 years)

Of these patients admitted to hospital with burns or scalds, males outnumber females by 2.6 to 1 and 75 per cent of the males are in the age group 15–44 years. These findings reflect the additional hazards of industrial injuries and of the accident proneness of younger workers. As might be expected, most of the serious industrial burns are caused by clothing catching fire, particularly in association with highly flammable liquids such as petrol (gasoline), paraffin (kerosine) and industrial solvents. The commonest type of burn, however, in this group of patients is a 'flash' injury caused either by the radiant heat of an electrical short-circuit or the transient flame of a gas or vapour explosion.

Elderly adults (65–85+ years)

Although the *total* incidence of burns and scalds per 10 000 population aged 65 years and over is almost equally divided between males and females, there is a much greater incidence of injury to females (1.44:1) in the 75–84 year group. Because females outnumber males by almost 2 to 1 in this age group and by over 3 to 1 in the 85+ group, females comprise 77 per cent of all patients aged 75+ admitted to hospital with burns and scalds.

Many of these injuries result from the general decline in balance, coordination and dexterity that accompanies old age, and falls onto fires and against hot surfaces, clothing brushing against naked flames and accidents with containers of hot liquids are common causes of thermal injury. In a significant proportion of cases, an event such as a stroke, heart attack or sudden loss of consciousness is the precipitating cause of the thermal injury.

Mortality

In 1983, there were 629 deaths from fire and flames in England and Wales, a decline of about 80 per cent since 1900. This dramatic reduction is due to a number of different factors, some inter-related and others quite separate from one another. Inter-related factors include changes in methods of heating and lighting the homes and the workplace, style and nature of clothing, an increasing awareness of the hazards of naked flames, legislation to improve the safety of heat sources and the flammability of certain types of clothing and health and safety legislation to reduce hazards at work. These changes, forming part of the social history of life and work in England and Wales since the beginning of the century, have resulted in a decrease in the incidence and severity of thermal injury.

At the same time, but quite separate from these social changes, there have been important advances in the methods of treating burns so that the mortality rate for some patients is now only a fraction of what it was in 1900. For instance, during the first quarter of this century, burn shock was ill understood and, consequently, effective intravenous fluid therapy was seldom provided. In these circumstances it must have been a rare event for any patient with an extensive burn to survive past the first few days. Between 1930 and 1955, the nature of the fluid shift in burns was elucidated and effective treatment based on intravenous infusion was developed and widely publicized. The advent of effective resuscitation ensured survival for many patients with moderately extensive burns, but for those with very large burns the tendency was for death to be deferred rather than prevented. It is not surprising, in retrospect, that when patients were able to survive past the first few days, the problems associated with the closure of these wounds of unprecedented size would not be solved immediately. In this group of patients, invasive sepsis was the most important cause of death and the history of burn patient care from the 1940s to the 1970s comprises a series of battles to overcome the pathogenic effects of the micro-organisms that colonized the burn wounds with consummate ease.

With the introduction of penicillin in the 1940s it became possible to control *Streptococcus pyogenes*, but the emergence of penicillinase-producing *Staphylococcus aureus* required the development of semisynthetic penicillins that were penicillinase resistant (e.g. methicillin, cloxacillin etc.) before an effective control of Gram-positive organisms was possible. During the 1950s and early 1960s the widespread and indiscriminate use of broad-spectrum antibiotics gave rise to a serious situation in which mortality rate was actually rising for patients with extensive burns who were now dying of Gram-negative septicaemia, *Pseudomonas aeruginosa* being the principal culprit. From 1965, better methods of controlling *Pseudomonas* sp. on the burn wound became available with the introduction of 0.5 per cent silver nitrate solution, sulfamylon and silver sulphadiazine. At the same time, the systemic use of gentamicin made possible for the first time the effective treatment of pseudomonas septicaemia. These improvements in antimicrobial therapy and other avances including better nutritional support and earlier and more efficient ways of closing the burn wound have improved the chances of survival for patients with extensive burns but, unfortunately, other factors related to thermal injury have had the opposite effect. In order to understand the significance of these changes, it is necessary to have a method of identifying the severity of a burn injury and thus some measure of how likely it is that the patient will survive, assuming that a good standard of specialized care is available. Such a measure is provided by deriving for each patient an index known as the 'mortality probability'.

Mortality probability

In 1954, Bull and Fisher described a statistical method that produced a mortality probability based on the outcome for 2807 patients treated in Birmingham in the 10-year period 1942–52. The number of deaths in this series had been 161 and it became clear that the principal determinants of whether a patient lived or died were the size of the burn and the age of the patient. In 1971, Bull published a revised mortality probability grid based on the additional information provided by a further series of 1922 patients admitted in the years 1965–70 and in which 122 deaths had occurred. This revised mortality probability grid is shown in *Table 1.1*. As Bull pointed out: 'As with previous similar charts it is important that this be used in retrospect to assess results for a group of patients rather than to judge the clinical prospects of an individual case which may well have a prognosis better or

Table 1.3 Mortality, all patients in Yorkshire Regional Burns Centre in 1966–83

Year	No of. patients	Deaths		Cause of death	
		Predicted No. (%)	Actual No. (%)	Septicaemia No. (%)	Smoke No. (%)
1966–71	419	60.7 (14.5)	59 (14.0)	11 (2.63)	4 (0.95)
1972–77	549	71.6 (13.0)	77 (18.5)	13 (2.37)	11 (2.00)
1978–83	461	87.7 (19.0)	93 (20.2)	9 (1.95)	22 (4.77)

'death from natural causes' (based on postmortem findings) was the cause of death recorded by HM Coroner. However, in reporting the outcome of the series of 1429 patients, these deaths are all counted as burn deaths and the category 'natural causes' is simply a convenient way of identifying a group of patients for whom the outcome would not have been affected by improvements in burn patient care.

Similarly, the second group – not actively resuscitated – comprises patients with massive unsurvivable burns most of whom were also very elderly. For these patients, mainly in the 70+ age group with burns of 60 per cent or more, a reduction in the number of deaths will come only by measures to prevent the burns occurring.

The two most important causes of death, where improvements in methods of treatment could lead to a reduction in mortality, are smoke inhalation and septicaemia. In *Table 1.3* the 1429 patients are subdivided into three consecutive 6-year periods. Although on the basis of overall mortality, it would seem that treatment in 1978–83 was no better than in 1966–71 and might even have been worse, examination of the numbers of deaths caused by septicaemia and smoke inhalation reveals a different picture. In 1966–71, death from septicaemia was 2.63 per cent whereas in 1973–83 the percentage was 1.95 – an 'improvement' that just fails to be statistically significant but is unlikely to represent a worse situation. At the same time, deaths from smoke inhalation had risen from 0.95 per cent in 1966–71 to 4.77 per cent in 1978–83 which is statistically highly significant ($P<0.01$). In other words, the lack of improvement in overall mortality is attributable to an increase in deaths from smoke inhalation; it is this change, of epidemic proportions, that caused the death of 10 per cent of all patients admitted during 1978–83 who had burns of 20 per cent or more.

There is general agreement amongst those who work in burn centres in the United Kingdom that deaths from smoke inhalation have increased enormously in recent years and are now the most important single cause of death in burn patients. Much of the problem results from the presence of plastics in all environments because, when these substances burn, they release large quantities of highly toxic or corrosive combustion products. For example, polyvinyl chloride (PVC) burns to produce, amongst other things, hydrochloric acid and phosgene. It is the highly corrosive effect of these gases upon the alveolar membrane which produces severe pulmonary damage that is difficult to treat. Perhaps the biggest irony is that, although smoke control legislation in the 1950s has, by taking away so many open fires, indirectly played an important part in reducing death, disability and disfigurement in a whole generation of young girls, some new form of 'smoke control legislation' is now required to stem the rising tide of deaths which result from inhaling the smoke of burning plastics.

Prevention

The personal tragedies involved in serious burning accidents need no elaboration. The cost to the community is high, involving in England and Wales some 60 000 patient-weeks of acute hospital care; the cost to the individual patient is often overwhelming. No scale of values can measure the immense suffering endured by patients with extensive burns: prolonged periods during which painful dressings have to be done every second day, blood transfusions accepted, gallons of high-protein feeds swallowed, and extensive and debilitating operations undergone; and often at the end of the illness, the prospect of further long programmes of plastic surgery to minimize the disability and disfigurement.

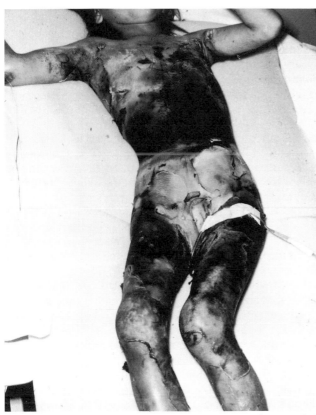

Figure 1.5 The tragic sight of a 5-year-old whose party dress caught fire, causing 65 per cent burns; she lived for 19 days

Most of the serious injuries are still due to clothing burns from domestic accidents involving unguarded fires and 90 per cent of deaths from domestic burns are due to ignition of clothing. It is in this area that preventive measures are hardest to implement although they would pay the greatest dividends. It is a civil offence in the United Kingdom to leave a child under the age of 12 alone in a house where any heating appliance is installed, but these regulations are not enforceable, and prosecutions are very seldom undertaken after an accident has occurred, the authorities being loath to cause further distress to relatives already supposedly sufficiently remorseful. Better manufacturer's standards for built-in guards on electric fires and gas-fires, enforced since 1952, have markedly reduced accidents from these sources, and with the encouragement of central heating systems to replace open fires as part of long-term antipollution measures, the total number of these injuries has decreased. Epileptic patients pose a special problem in this respect, as almost always when injured they are found to have neglected to take their anticonvulsant pills, and have had an inadequately guarded fire. There may have been a fireguard, but unless it is fixed to the chimney-breast, it will collapse if the victim falls against it during a seizure. Only repeated sympathetic advice from the family doctor can have any effect in these special cases (Tempest, 1970).

The other main avenue of attack on the problem, applicable to industrial countries, is the wider application of flame-proofing of textiles generally, and to clothing in particular. The first legislation limiting the sale of highly flammable textiles was passed in the USA in 1954. Since that time officially authorized test methods must be complied with before a fabric can be offered for sale, and similar standards are enforced in Switzerland and some other countries. In the United Kingdom, the sale of highly flammable children's nightwear was prohibited in 1964 and, in addition, since 1967 adult nightwear which has not passed the slow combustion test laid down in British Standard BS 3121 has to be so labelled by the manufacturer.

There is no doubt that the development of flame-retardant nightwear has been of importance in the reduction of serious burns to girls, but fire-guard regulations, a change in fashion from nightdresses to pyjamas and the general reduction in the number of open fires have all contributed to the fall in clothing-related injuries. Although the Nightdresses (Safety) Regulations require children's nightdresses to satisfy the requirements of the British Standard BS 3121, some pressure is developing for these regulations to be extended to include pyjamas and dressing gowns. However, perhaps the most that can be achieved in the near future is for all nightwear, including pyjamas, to have easily seen labels that indicate whether or not they are flammable.

Flammability is dependent upon several factors: the kind of fibre or plastic, the type of fabric construction and its openness or tightness and weight, the style and decorative features, and the nature of the immediate environment. Ideally, all fabrics sold should be flame resistant, but it must be remembered that such fabrics are expensive to produce and have undesirable effects on handle and drape if they are to be fast to repeated washing. For commercial reasons this prevents a large number of fabrics from being given a flame-resistant treatment. An 'all or nothing' attitude on the part of those who are concerned with prevention of burns would be counterproductive; the aim should be to encourage the manufacture of fabrics which are no more flammable than wool, for which no one would consider fireproofing necessary for clothing purposes.

Cotton, flannelette (fluffed cotton) and rayon (extruded cellulose) are all flammable unless treated. Wool and real silk burn poorly. Nylon, Terylene and similar synthetic materials burn poorly if directly ignited, but melt when caught in the flame of other burning fabrics. Some large stores have led and still lead the way by not stocking articles of children's wear that they consider to be dangerous.

By contrast with clothing burns, scalds in children are fortunately seldom fatal, but they are painful and often result in disfigurement. Accidents involving electric kettles are responsible for many of the more serious scalds in young children, typically as a consequence of the child pulling on the kettle flex as it hangs over the worktop. Coiled electric kettle flexes are now available that minimize this danger, and their more general use would reduce the incidence of these injuries. With regard to other aspects of kettle design, spout-filling kettles, when upturned, spill their contents less easily than those with lids, and most of the newer 'jug-shaped' kettles are more easily knocked over (and spill their contents more quickly) than kettles of traditional design. Manufacturers should be encouraged to improve the safety of their products where this is possible.

All these measures are helpful in reducing the number of burning accidents, and in mitigating their severity, and further slow but steady progress is to be expected. The differing scales of the problem of burn prevention in less developed areas of the world than western Europe are outside the scope of this book.

Doctors and hospital workers generally could help a great deal by taking accurate notes of all burning accidents: what the circumstances were when it happened, what type of clothing the victim was wearing, and what first aid was applied. There is a great need for all accidents involving burns, those requiring admission to hospital and those requiring significant out-patient treatment, to be properly recorded in a manner which makes for easy retrieval. McQueen (1960) found that 10 patients with burns or scalds required out-patient treatment for each one admitted to hospital, and that half of these were off work for three days or more. If the real size of the problem of burns injuries (as opposed to the deaths only) was accurately known, the economic and social costs could be assessed, and a proper proportion of funds and resources allocated for both the prevention and the treatment of these serious injuries.

References

BULL, J. P. (1971) Revised analysis of mortality due to burns. *Lancet*, **ii**, 1133–1134

BULL, J. P. and FISHER, A. J. (1954) A study of mortality in burns: a revised estimate. *Annals of Surgery*, **139**, 269

DEPARTMENT OF HEALTH AND SOCIAL SECURITY (1981) *Hospital In-Patient Enquiry*. Series MB4, No. 17, HMSO

DEPARTMENT OF TRADE (1983) *Domestic Thermal Injuries. A Study of 1100 Accidents admitted to Specialised Treatment Centres*. Department of Trade (now Department of Trade and Industry)

McQUEEN, I. A. G. (1960) *A Study of Home Accidents in Aberdeen*. Edinburgh: E. & S. Livingstone

MOORES, B., RAHMAN, M. M., BROWNING, F. S. C. and SETTLE, J. A. D. (1975) Discriminant function analysis of 570 consecutive burns patients admitted to the Yorkshire Regional Burns Centre between 1966 and 1973. *Burns*, **1**, 135–141

TEMPEST, M. (1970) Burns in epileptic patients: a survey of admissions to a regional Burns Centre over a twenty-year period. In *Research In Burns: Transactions of the Third International Congress on Research in Burns*, Eds P. Malter, T. L. Barclay and Z. Konickova, Prague 1970, p. 54. Bern: Hans Huber

Chapter 2

Treatment of burns shock

Following a severe burn the patient may pass into a state of shock, and it is the recognition and management of this condition which is the surgeon's most urgent duty during the first few days after such an injury.

Primary shock

Primary shock occurs immediately after burning, and is similar to that occurring after other painful injuries. Primary shock passes off spontaneously, and is rarely still present by the time that a doctor first sees the patient. No specific treatment is indicated for this condition, and it will not be discussed further.

Secondary shock

During the first few hours after the burn the patient passes gradually into the stage of secondary shock, and all subsequent discussion refers to this phenomenon. The discussion is divided into five sections for ease of reference:

(*a*) Pathology.
(*b*) Background considerations of treatment.
(*c*) The practical management of burns shock.
(*d*) Other methods of treatment.
(*e*) Complications during the shock period.

Pathology of burns shock

At the surface of the burn a greater or lesser depth of the skin is actually destroyed by the heat, but immediately underneath this destroyed tissue the deeper layers of the skin and the subcutaneous tissue are severely affected by the heat, but still viable. In these layers the main changes are in the capillaries which become widely dilated and of greatly increased permeability. The increased permeability causes a disturbance in the normal exchange of fluid between the blood plasma and the extracellular space, and fluid is rapidly lost from the plasma into the extracellular space at the site of the burn. When this fluid is lost into the skin it appears as blisters if the skin surface remains intact, or as an exudate from the raw surface if the outer layers of skin are lost. When the fluid is lost into the subcutaneous tissue it causes oedematous swelling. The fluid lost from the plasma in this way contains electrolytes in the same concentrations as in the plasma, and an amount of protein which varies from one burn to another, and also varies in different parts of the same burn.

It has often been stated that the protein content of the exudate is half that of the blood plasma, but during the critical first 24 hours it is invariably higher, and of the order of 80 per cent of the level in the blood plasma.

Differential analysis of the various proteins of the exudate shows that the proportions are approximately the same as those in blood plasma, although there is usually a relative preponderance of the smaller albumin molecules.

The typical findings in blister fluid from a burn of moderate severity are:

Plasma		*Blister fluid*	
Total protein	6.5 g %	Total protein	5.0 g %
Albumin	3.9 g %	Albumin	3.7 g %
Globulin	2.6 g %	Globulin	1.3 g %

Sometimes clotting occurs in blister fluid showing that the large fibrinogen molecules (molecular weight 400 000) have passed through the capillary walls and, in the patient whose figures are shown above, it was possible to demonstrate the presence of anti-B red cell agglutinins in the blister fluid (probable molecular weight 900 000).

In other instances, the capillary walls become so incompetent that a diapedesis of red corpuscles occurs, and this can often be seen in deep partial thickness burns, when it causes a characteristic red and white mottling which cannot be affected by pressure.

The loss of fluid from the circulation continues at a rapid rate for some hours, and then gradually decreases over the course of one to two days as the capillaries recover their tone and permeability, and reabsorption of the oedema fluid begins to take place. The amount of oedema that occurs depends partly upon the circumstances of the burn, i.e. the temperature and time of exposure, and partly upon the elasticity and tissue tension of the part affected. Thus, in the face where the tissues are relatively lax and easily distensible the swelling will be great and obvious, while in places with a high tissue elasticity, such as the limbs, much less swelling will occur.

The loss of this protein-rich fluid from the plasma at the site of the burn is the factor of over-riding importance in the causation of the clinical condition of shock in burned patients. The fluid loss results in a fall in plasma volume and, because there is proportionately less loss of protein than electrolyte solution, there occurs a slight rise in plasma osmotic pressure. The natural defence reaction of the body is to counteract this fall of plasma volume in three ways:

(a) By withdrawing fluid from the undamaged part of the extracellular space probably under the influence of the raised osmotic pressure, but possibly due to other causes also.

(b) By a general constriction of blood vessels in the splanchnic area and the skin. This constriction of vessels reduces the space which the available blood volume has to fill, and increases the peripheral resistance so that the blood pressure is maintained, and an adequate blood supply to the vital organs is continued. It was originally thought that the vascular changes were due mainly to sympathetic nervous activity, but it now seems more likely that circulatory catecholamines are more important and increased activity of the renin–angiotensin system may also be involved.

(c) By ingestion and absorption of fluid from the gut in response to a feeling of thirst.

By these mechanisms the body may be able to compensate adequately for the fluid loss and, when the rate of loss of fluid is not too great, i.e. in less severe burns, the patient may pass safely through the phase of shock with no other help than the provision of extra fluid to drink. By 36 hours after the injury, the damaged capillaries will recover their tone and permeability, reabsorption of fluid from the interstitial space at the site of the burn will occur, and the danger of shock will be over.

When the burn is more severe, however, and the rate of loss is more rapid, the plasma volume continues to fall. The degree of splanchnic vasoconstriction becomes more intense until the visceral blood flow is reduced to a dangerously low level. The most obvious effects are on the kidney and intestine. The urine output falls to a very low level or even to zero, indicating a very poor renal blood flow, and in a short time the cells of the kidney may be so damaged by anoxia that they may fail to recover even if the blood flow is subsequently raised to normal levels.

In the intestine, constriction of the arterioles may be so intense that the blood flow is inadequate to satisfy the needs of the cells of the capillary walls, and the capillaries become anoxic, passively dilated and incapable of functioning. Absorption of fluid from the intestine cannot occur, peristalsis ceases, and if the patient, who is by now intensely thirsty, attempts to drink he will vomit.

The patient has now become the victim of a vicious circle, and the very defence mechanism, which in the early stages could compensate for the fall in blood volume, has now become harmful and will prevent the patient from restoring his blood volume by natural means, i.e. by absorption of fluid from the gut.

At the same time as these events are going on in the viscera, a similar sequence of events takes place in the skin. This is initially pale because the capillaries as well as the arterioles are contracted; but the arteriolar constriction may become so intense that the capillary walls themselves become anoxic, the capillaries can no longer contract and passively dilate filling slowly with blood which becomes de-oxygenated, and gives the characteristic blue-grey colour to the skin. Even at this stage, however, the peripheral blood pressure may still be kept up by the compensating vasoconstriction, and the blood flow to the brain is maintained to the last, so that consciousness is lost late.

Loss of red cells

So far we have discussed only the loss of plasma from the circulation and, indeed, this overshadows all other factors in its importance. In some burns, however, red blood cells may also be lost in sufficient numbers to cause substantial falls in total red cell volume, and the effect of this will be to intensify the effect of plasma loss. It has been known for many years that patients with severe burns may show free haemoglobin in the plasma and urine, indicating that red cells have been haemolysed by heat at the time of the burn, and in other patients unexpectedly low haemoglobin concentrations after the shock period indicate that considerable loss of red cells has occurred. It is known that this loss of red cells is associated only with deep burns and not with superficial burns, and some years ago it became accepted that all extensive deep burns were associated with substantial loss of red cells, and that these patients required whole blood transfusions during the shock period (Evans and Biggar, 1945; Kyle and Wallace, 1951; Moyer, 1953). Improved methods of total red cell volume estimations, however, have shown that the loss of red cells is usually gradual, and not as severe as was originally thought (Davies and Topley, 1956; Topley and Jackson, 1957; Muir, 1961). The loss of red cells during the shock period falls into three distinct phases:

(*a*) A number of red cells are actually destroyed by heat at the time of the burn, and if the quantity destroyed is sufficient this will become manifest as obvious haemoglobinaemia and haemoglobinuria.

(*b*) A number of red cells not destroyed by heat at the time of the burn are rendered abnormally fragile, and these are removed within the first few hours by the reticuloendothelial system (*Figure 2.1*)

   The loss of red cells from these two causes is proportional to the severity of the burn, but even in deep burns of up to 50 per cent of the body area, this loss does not usually exceed 10 per cent of the total red cell volume.

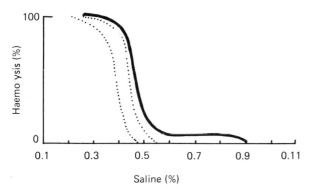

Figure 2.1 The saline fragility curve of blood from a patient hours after a severe 30 per cent burn. Note the 'tail' indicating that 10 per cent of the cells are very fragile and will soon be removed from the circulation. The main body of the curve is to the right of normal limits, indicating a general increase of fragility of the cells

(*c*) During the main part of the shock period red cell loss continues for causes unknown. Evidence indicates that the cells are not lost into the burnt skin, but that for some reason they are prematurely removed by the reticuloendothelial system, although the fragility curves at this stage do not show evidence of unusual fragility. The loss during this important stage bears no relationship to the size of the burn, but again does not usually exceed one-tenth of the red cell volume in burns of up to 50 per cent of the body area. A few patients, however, lose larger volumes of red cells of the order of one-quarter of the total red cell volume, and occasionally still larger volumes of red cells may be lost, thus causing serious difficulties with treatment (*see* p. 45).

Electrolyte changes

The large volumes of fluid which move from one compartment to another in burns shock are associated with corresponding shifts of electrolytes, since the electrolyte content of the fluid is similar to that of the normal blood plasma and interstitial fluid. In some cases, however, in addition to the shifts, there is a fall in the sodium content of the extracellular fluid. This appears to be due to two causes. Damaged collagen in the burned area absorbs sodium selectively and the membranes of damaged cells allow sodium to leak into the cells and potassium to diffuse out. These changes are usually slight and if the circulatory defect is corrected there is a gradual return to normal values. However, if the blood volume defect is allowed to persist this will lead ultimately to more serious abnormalities at the cellular level and in the interstitial fluid.

Sometimes, even in apparently well-treated patients, changes in the cell membranes may give rise to serious abnormalities of intracellular electrolytes which cannot be deduced from examination of the plasma electrolytes. These changes characteristically occur late in the shock period or some days after the shock period is over and are responsible for the so-called 'sick-cell' syndrome which is discussed later.

The background considerations of the treatment of burns shock by replacement transfusion

The progression of a patient from compensated to uncompensated shock and finally to a gross hypotensive state has been described and the aims of treatment of shock can now be stated.

The surgeon's task is to recognize at the outset those patients who will be unable to make good the fluid loss by natural means and are therefore liable to pass into a state of uncompensated shock and to treat them by intravenous infusion of appropriate fluids so that the blood volume is never allowed to fall below the critical level at which the defence mechanisms become harmful. In this way an adequate blood flow to the vulnerable viscera is ensured until reabsorption of fluid at the site of the burn takes place and the danger of shock is over.

It should be emphasized that the aim of treatment by transfusion should be prevention, rather than cure, of the uncompensated state. The surgeon should keep always one step ahead of the developing condition. Burns shock differs from other forms of traumatic shock inasmuch as its relatively slow development over a period of hours enables the compensating mechanism of splanchnic vasoconstriction to develop fully and this mechanism, while keeping up the blood pressure, may itself result in severe and irreversible damage to the kidney or other viscera. Actual hypotension which occurs late in efficiently treated cases must not be allowed to develop.

Patients requiring transfusion

Studies of the clinical histories of large numbers of patients have shown that the amount of loss of fluid varies with the surface area of skin involved by burning, but that the amount of fluid lost for comparable areas of skin is similar irrespective of the depth of burning, a relatively superficial burn resulting in as much fluid loss as a deeper one. Furthermore, it has been possible to establish the critical area of burning below which the patient can compensate for loss of fluid by natural means, and above which he is liable to go into uncontrolled, uncompensated shock unless assisted by transfusion. It has been found that this critical area is 15 per cent of the body surface in adults, but that children tolerate the loss of fluid less well, and can only withstand burns of less than 10 per cent of the body surface by natural means (Gibson and Brown, 1945; Kyle and Wallace, 1951).

It follows, therefore, that adults with burns of less than 15 per cent and children with burns of less than 10 per cent surface area can be treated simply by the administration of extra fluids by mouth, and that transfusion will not be required. With burns larger than these sizes, however, it is known that shock is likely to develop, and transfusion should therefore be started as soon as possible, and continued until the danger of shock is over.

Type of fluid to be used for transfusion

The composition of the fluid lost from the plasma has already been described; it is generally agreed to be of normal electrolyte content and contains about 5 g of protein per 100 ml. There is, however, considerable disagreement about the relative importance of the loss of the various constituents from the plasma and consequently about the type of fluid which should be transfused. Comparison between blood plasma, burn blister fluid, and different preparations for intravenous use is shown in *Figure 2.2*. Plasma, plasma substitutes, and various electrolyte solutions all have their advocates. Saline was the fluid first used for intravenous infusion in burns, but when plasma became available this was generally preferred because it resembled more closely the fluid lost from the circulation and was believed to produce better results. On the frequently noted (but in our view erroneous) grounds that burn fluid contains half the protein content of normal plasma, some workers suggested that the transfused fluid should consist of equal volumes of dried reconstituted plasma and normal saline. As the protein content of dried plasma is only 5 g/100 ml it can be seen that this gives an effective concentration of only 2.5 g/100 ml which we believe to be inadequate (Batchelor, Kirk and Sutherland, 1961). Subsequent workers reduced the proportion of plasma in the transfusion still further and claimed that equally satisfactory results could be obtained if the plasma:saline ratio was as low as one-third or even one-quarter (Reiss *et al.*, 1953; Artz and Reiss, 1957).

Over the last 15 years there has been a further swing away from the use of plasma (and other colloids) and in the majority of countries at the present time shock treatment is by Ringer–lactate (Hartmanns') solution or some other electrolyte solution. The reasons for this are not wholly on grounds of clinical choice and it is clear that consideration of cost has much influence.

Electrolyte solutions are cheap and readily available (80 pence for a 500-ml bottle) whereas plasma is expensive (£50 per 500 ml) and is quite unobtainable in many countries. The experience of many excellent centres has shown that electrolyte transfusion can give results which are comparable if not identical with the results of plasma transfusion and, when financial factors are predominant, then electrolyte treatment is obviously acceptable.

Much effort has been expended in comparing the results of treatment, usually in an attempt to decide if one method is 'better' than the other. The literature contains a huge number of reports of animal experiments which were designed to answer this question, but it must be stated at once that, without exception, the circumstances and techniques of animal experiments bear no relationship to the circumstances and techniques of treatment of human patients and the results of the animal experiments can be applied to clinical practice only with the strictest

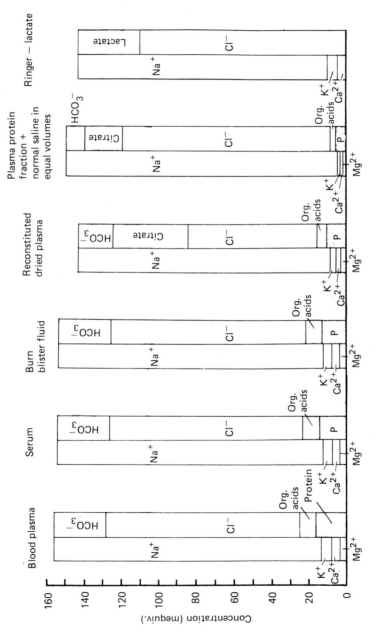

Figure 2.2 The comparison between burn blister fluid and various types of fluid used for transfusion

reservations. Of much more importance are the clinical studies of large groups of patients treated by different methods (Markley *et al.*, 1956; Jackson and Cason, 1966; Masterton and Dudley, 1971). These studies suggest that the overall mortality differs little between patients treated by plasma or by electrolytes, but it is clear that there are important differences in the physiological behaviour of patients treated by the two methods and these must be understood if confusion is to be avoided.

It is believed that the present evidence indicates that transfusion by plasma in optimal amounts gives at least as good a result as treatment by other methods. Furthermore, by using plasma it is possible to keep more of the body's functions closer to normal than by any other method and the circumstantial evidence indicates that this is desirable. Reconstituted dried human plasma resembles closely the fluid lost from the circulation at the site of the burn and replacement of this lost fluid is theoretically most consistent with our concept of burn shock as an oligaemic shock due to diminished plasma volume.

Consideration must, however, be given to the increasing difficulty of obtaining whole plasma. There is such a need for different blood products that there is strong pressure on the Blood Transfusion Service to fractionate plasma donations so as to remove and separate the larger protein molecules – globulins, fibrinogen etc. – thus leaving a solution containing only albumin and electrolytes, the so-called 'plasma protein solution' (PPS) or 'plasma protein fraction' (PPF). This is now offered in place of plasma and, since the burns departments in the UK have had insufficient opportunity to demonstrate that whole plasma has a significant advantage over the albumin solution, it seems likely that this is the only form of 'plasma' which will be available for the future.

The method of treatment using this plasma protein solution is described first and then any disadvantages are considered followed by description of alternative methods of treatment.

It is recommended that the basic fluid for replacement therapy should be 'plasma protein solution' because, of the fluids readily available in this country at the moment, this resembles most closely the fluid lost from the circulation at the site of the burn.

In the past a serious disadvantage has been the possibility of transmission of the virus of hepatitis but all donated blood is now screened for Australia antigen and only antigen-free donors are accepted.

The emergence of AIDS (Acquired Immune Deficiency Syndrome) and its transmission by means of blood products has produced a new problem. However all blood donors are now screened for AIDS antibody and in addition plasma protein solution is heat treated to destroy any possible infective agent.

Clinical signs

The aim of transfusion is to maintain the blood volume at a sufficient level to ensure an adequate blood supply to the vital organs and particularly to the viscera.

What objectives should be kept in mind, and what are the indications that the transfusion is being successful?

The signs of value for determining the adequacy of transfusion fall into three groups:

(*a*) Signs indicating the state of the circulation in general:
    (i)   Presence or absence of restlessness.

      (ii)   Colour of skin.
     (iii) Superficial and deep body temperature.
     (iv) Blood pressure and pulse rate.
     (v)   Central venous pressure (CVP), and pulmonary artery pressure.

(*b*) Signs indicating the state of the visceral circulation:
     (vi) Urine output – volume and concentration.
    (vii) Absorption of fluid by the gut.

(*c*) Guides to plasma volume:
   (viii) Haematocrit or haemoglobin concentration of peripheral blood.

Restlessness
This is an important sign particularly in children. Restlessness is usually indicative of oligaemia, although sometimes other factors are responsible and a distressed child may still be restless even with adequate transfusion. The child who goes quietly off to sleep and is obviously restful is certainly in a good state.

The colour of the skin
The circulation in the skin to some extent reflects that in the internal organs, and examination of the skin therefore gives a valuable clue to progress. Pink skin indicates dilated arterioles and capillaries, and shows that the circulation is certainly adequate. Pallor of the skin is usually a good sign indicating contracted capillaries but with still enough blood flow for the capillaries to remain active. In severely shocked patients, however, the skin becomes a bluish-grey colour indicating stagnation of blood in maximally dilated capillaries, and this is invariably a bad sign.

    Marked coldness of the tip of the nose is also an unfavourable sign which is easily discerned.

Skin and deep body temperature
The temperature of the skin can readily be measured by a thermistor probe attached to a toe and the difference between this reading and the deep body temperature, as measured by a probe in the rectum or the external auditory meatus, gives good confirmation of the degree of peripheral vasoconstriction. Initially the difference may be large and a gradual narrowing of the gap is confirmatory evidence of improvement.

Blood pressure and pulse rate
It has already been pointed out that fall in blood pressure is a late manifestation of burns shock and is an indication that the surgeon has fallen far behind in his replacement programme. Proper attention to the other signs usually makes blood pressure readings redundant and when, in severely burned patients, it is impossible to find a suitable length of unburned limb round which the blood pressure cuff can be applied, there should be no hesitation in omitting routine blood pressure readings.

    The pulse rate will be recorded as part of the routine nursing procedures. The rate is subjected to so many influences that changes from hour to hour are of little significance. A gradual fall from a high rate towards normal gives minor confirmatory evidence of improving circulation.

Central venous pressure
Measurement of central venous pressure (CVP) has been extensively used during the treatment of shock, particularly in accident surgery and during major operations. It is particularly useful when haemodynamic changes are occurring rapidly. In burns shock, however, the haemodynamic changes occur more gradually and it is usually possible to maintain satisfactory control without the use of CVP measurements. It should be remembered that in burned patients there is a greater likelihood of infection entering the blood stream along the track of the CVP catheter than in most other shocked patients: it may, for instance, be impossible to introduce the catheter except through an area of burned skin. The authors believe, therefore, that CVP measurements should not be made as a routine but only when consideration of the other signs leaves doubt as to the adequacy of fluid replacements.

CVP measurements are particularly valuable in the assessment of patients with low urine output, and are essential if severe renal impairment has occurred. This problem is discussed below.

Pulmonary artery pressure
Some authorities consider that the pulmonary artery pressure (so-called pulmonary wedge pressure) as measured by a Swan–Ganz catheter is a more reliable measure of the state of the circulation than the CVP (Aikawa, Martyn and Burke, 1978). However, this involves a complicated technique which is difficult to apply in severely burned patients and it is likely to be a practical proposition only in exceptional circumstances.

Urine output
Of all the viscera, the kidney is the one most likely to be damaged by uncontrolled shock; it is fortunate that in the secretion of urine we have a valuable guide to the function and indirectly, therefore, to the blood flow of the kidney.

In the early stages after any injury, the kidney is subjected to intense activity by circulating catecholamines, angiotensin and by the antidiuretic hormones of the posterior pituitary (Le Quesne, 1957). Because of variability in these stimuli, changes in urine flow can be difficult to interpret. Some authorities, observing an apparent unpredictability and wide variation in hourly urine volumes, have concluded that urine volume is a totally unreliable index of the effectiveness of resuscitation (Barton and Laing, 1970) whilst others have used hourly urine volume as the main guide to infusion therapy (Baxter, 1971). It is our experience that to make any sense of urine output, the hourly urine volume and its concentration must be considered *together*, consequently both should be measured.

It is reasonable to assume that, following the occurrence of a burn large enough to require intravenous fluid therapy, antidiuretic hormone (ADH) will be present in the circulation for most of the first 24 hours. During this time water diuresis will not be possible and the urine will remain significantly more concentrated than the glomerular filtrate, i.e. urine osmolarity will be two or three times greater than the normal plasma osmolarity of around 300 mosmol/l. This persistent antidiuresis does not mean that the hourly urine volume will inevitably be very small because antidiuresis and oliguria are not synonymous; the former describes the concentration, the latter describes the volume. Indeed, it is in precisely the circumstances of maximal ADH activity that a direct linear relationship exists between total solute excretion and urine volume. Hence, an increase in filtered solute load, whether resulting from an increased glomerular filtration rate or from the presence of a disposable solute such as glucose, mannitol or low-molecular-weight dextran, will promote an increased urine volume but with *an inverse fall in its concentration*. (It is *possible* for water diuresis to occur even within the first 8 hours following a major burn (Settle, 1974), but it is usually a transient response to a dangerously large water load that has depressed plasma osmolarity below 275 mosmol/l – a hazardous situation that should be avoided by limiting the sodium-free water intake of the patient.)

In the absence of a large amount of disposable solute (glucose, mannitol etc.) in the glomerular filtrate and the avoidance of a massive sodium-free water intake, the final urine will be significantly concentrated (600–900 mosmol/l) compared with the glomerular filtrate *unless serious impairment of renal function occurs*. If the doctor is certain that a concentrated urine is being produced, urine flow is a useful index of effective resuscitation. In these circumstances, a satisfactory flow rate is 0.5–1.0 ml/h per kg body weight, e.g. an hourly volume of 35–70 ml for an adult patient (Settle, 1974). An hourly volume below 0.5 ml/h per kg, with a concentration above 800 mosmol/l is a reliable indication that infusion therapy is inadequate, while volumes well over 1.0 ml/h per kg, with a concentration of 350–450 mosmol/l strongly indicate over-transfusion.

Measurement of urine volume   A closed urinary drainage system should be connected to the indwelling catheter. The design should permit the accurate measurement of each hour's urine output and allow a small sample of that output to be removed without risk of bacterial contamination of the drainage system.

Measurement of urine concentration   The time-honoured way of estimating urine concentration is by measuring specific gravity, i.e. the ratio of the density of the urine to that of pure water at 4 °C. Thus, specific gravity is an index of the weight of solute present in the urine. However, the biologically significant aspect of a urine's concentration is its osmotic potential or osmolarity, which is a consequence of the *number* of particles of solute in solution and not the *weight* of these particles. Because of this, it is possible for urines of identical osmolarity to have widely different specific gravities as a consequence of solutes such as glucose or protein being present in differing amounts. The truth of this may be seen from the fact that 0.9 per cent saline (280 mosmol/l) has a specific gravity of 1.006 whilst 5 per cent glucose solution (280 mosmol/l) has a specific gravity of 1.019. (Even greater discrepancies occur if refractive index is used as an indicator of urine concentration. Instances have been seen where urine with an osmolarity of 350 mosmol/l has given 'specific gravity' readings as high as 1.030 when 'measured' in a urine refractometer.)

If at all possible, urine concentration should be determined by measurement of urine osmolarity. Using a depression of freezing point method, this measurement can be performed on a sample as small as 0.2 ml and takes only two minutes. It has been routine in the Yorkshire Regional Burns Centre since 1969 and, in recent years, has been performed by the nursing staff as each hourly urine is collected. Measurement of urine urea concentration and determination of urine:blood urea ratio provide an estimate of renal concentrating power that is useful in the diagnosis of renal failure, but any pathology laboratory that is capable of measuring urea concentration of hourly samples would almost certainly offer osmolarity measurement as a better alternative.

Interpreting the urine output   It is most useful to plot the values for urine flow rate and osmolarity as graphs, one above the other, just as pulse rate and temperature are conventionally charted. When volume and concentration can be seen at a glance, the inverse relationship between them is obvious and the trends from hour to hour can easily be seen. Trends are much more important than single hourly values. For instance, a sharp fall in urine volume after several hours of adequate volumes of concentrated urine, particularly if the concentration of the small urine volume is similar to those of previous hours, is almost certainly a drainage problem rather than an indication of inadequate resuscitation or impairment of renal function. On the other hand, a gradual reduction of volume to barely adequate levels, with a reciprocal progressive rise in concentration, is clear evidence that fluid infusion should be increased. (Other patterns will be described later in the section on renal failure.)

Haemoglobin and haematocrit of the peripheral blood
The haematocrit of the peripheral blood is a measure of the proportions of circulating plasma and red cells. Because of the loss of plasma the haematocrit is invariably raised in the early stages of burns shock, and the level of the haematocrit gives a valuable guide to the state of the plasma volume. When the haematocrit is raised then the interpretation clearly is that the plasma volume is low. Since the haematocrit is only a ratio and not an absolute value, it does not always follow that a normal or low haematocrit indicates an adequate plasma volume, for the haematocrit is also affected by changes in the red cells, and with a pre-existing anaemia or after severe red cell destruction a low or normal haematocrit may exist with a plasma volume (and therefore a total blood volume) which is very much below normal.

In the early work on plasma transfusion in Glasgow (Gibson and Brown, 1945), the haematocrit was the principal factor used in deciding the rate and volume of the transfusion which was adjusted so as to bring the haematocrit to normal. It is certainly true that in many cases it is necessary to bring the haematocrit to, or nearly to, normal in order to achieve a satisfactory urinary output and gut function, but it is felt that the haematocrit should be only one of the factors to be taken into consideration in assessing the patient's condition and that the achievement of a normal haematocrit should not be regarded as an aim in itself irrespective of other considerations. In this connection it should be noted that the gradual return of haematocrit towards normal is often a more valuable sign than the actual level at any particular time.

It is usually impracticable to obtain frequent venous samples in burned patients, but serial estimations of the haematocrit or haemoglobin of blood from a skin prick give valuable evidence and should always be done. Our own preference is for a capillary tube haematocrit estimation using heparinized tubes and a high-speed centrifuge,* but a haemoglobin estimation using a photo-electric meter is

* Hawkesley high-speed micro-haematocrit.

satisfactory, and even the simple Sahli method is not to be despised. It is of advantage if the surgeon himself can perform the estimation in or near the ward rather than have to send specimens to a distant laboratory with consequent delay in obtaining the result. Actual plasma and red cell volume measurements have been used in research studies, but the methods are far too complicated and time consuming for routine use.

Rate of loss of fluid and the use of formulae

The rate of loss of fluid from the circulation is maximal over the first few hours, and then gradually declines over the course of the next one to two days, although occasionally in severe burns the loss may be prolonged into the third day, and the transfusion must be planned so as to keep pace with this changing rate of loss. Although the transfusion must be tailored to fit each individual case, it is of great value to have some idea at the outset of treatment what sort of volume and rate of transfusion are likely to be required, and for this reason many retrospective studies have been made of the volumes of fluid required by patients with burns of different sizes. These studies have resulted in the devising of various formulae for working out in advance the volume of transfusion fluid likely to be necessary for a particular patient.

The investigations have shown that the rate and volume of fluid loss *increases with increasing size of the area burned* and that, within fairly wide limits, the *loss of fluid is not related to the depth of the burn*; fluid is lost with comparable rapidity from all burns of greater severity than simple erythema. Clearly, also, the actual volume of fluid lost in, for instance, a 30 per cent surface area burn in an adult will be different from the volume lost in a child with a 30 per cent burn, and most of the recent formulae are based on the estimates of the percentage area of the burn and the weight of the patient. A formula based on surface area might be more accurate, but those based on size as judged by weight are accurate enough for practical use.

Early formulae were produced by Harkins (1942), and by the National Research Council of America (1943), and were followed by those of Cope and Moore (1947), E. I. Evans *et al.* (1952), Wallace (1953). These formulae have been of great value, but all suffer from the disadvantage that volumes are worked out to represent fluid requirements over unduly long periods. In practice this causes two difficulties. In the first place if it is found necessary to alter the rate of transfusion because of unsatisfactory clinical progress, the mathematics become unnecessarily complicated and, secondly, the very fact that they are worked out over these long periods fosters the impression that a patient can be transfused in accordance with a formula which is unlikely to require alteration, and takes the emphasis off the need for repeated clinical examination which we believe to be of vital importance.

In the authors view, the necessary qualities of a formula are that it should:

(*a*) Give an initial rate for starting off the transfusion.
(*b*) Be capable of being easily altered at frequent and suitable intervals in the light of clinical progress.
(*c*) Provide a basis for decreasing the rate of transfusion as the rate of loss decreases.

In order to keep pace as closely as possible with the rate of loss the transfusion should theoretically be changed frequently, say at least every hour. In practice this is neither necessary nor desirable, and it has been found satisfactory to change the rate of transfusion every 12 hours.

Trials were made at Mount Vernon Hospital of a number of different schemes and the following plan was finally chosen, and has been in use for a number of years.

The formula is planned so as to give equal volumes of fluid in six successive periods of 4, 4, 4, 6, 6, and 12 hours. *Figure 2.3* shows a block graph representing the fluid given if the volume originally worked out by the formula proves to be satisfactory and no alteration is required.

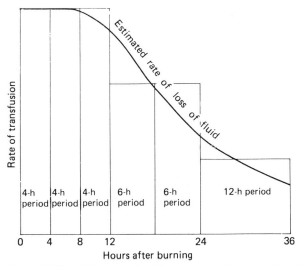

Figure 2.3 The thick curved line illustrates how the rate of loss of fluid from the circulation probably changes. The blocks represent equal volumes of transfusion fluid and show how the rate of transfusion is altered by varying the time during which the equal 'rations' are given

It can be seen that the rate of transfusion alters every 12 hours, and the slope of the graph of transfusion follows approximately the graph of probable rate of loss.

In practice only the fluid 'ration' for the first 4-hour period is worked out in the first instance on the basis of size of patient and area involved in burning, and this amount of fluid is transfused by the end of the *fourth hour after burning*. The drip is usually up about two hours after the injury, and this 'ration' will therefore be actually delivered in about two hours. At the end of this an assessment is made of the state of the patient and, if the amount is judged to have been adequate, the same volume is given in the next 4-hour period. If the assessment shows an unsatisfactory state, however, the plasma 'ration' for the second 4-hour period is altered accordingly. At the end of the second period the same procedure of assessment and working out of the 'ration' for the next period is made, and so on for each subsequent period.

The first period and to a lesser extent the second period are very much in the nature of trials, and the ends of these periods, which will usually come at two hours and six hours after the start of the transfusion, are good times for assessment. If, however, the burn is very severe, and anxiety is felt, assessments can be made more frequently and the transfusion altered accordingly.

The formula recommended for the *first period of four hours* is:

$$\frac{(\text{Total percentage of burn} \times \text{weight in kg})}{2} = \text{ml of fluid required.}$$

Cope and Moore (1947) investigated the expansion of the interstitial space in patients treated by transfusion of plasma and saline in equal proportions. They concluded that it is dangerous if the interstitial space expands by more than 50 per cent of its original size and, therefore, advised that when using a body weight/percentage area formula, body weight multiplied by 50 per cent should be the limiting factor irrespective of the size of the burn. Their reasoning is not easy to follow, as the transfusions in their patients appeared to be very much larger than would be indicated by their own formula. It should be noted that with the techniques these workers used it was not possible to differentiate between the affected interstitial space at the site of the burn and the unaffected part elsewhere. Other workers have similarly suggested that it is necessary to limit the volume of the transfusion to some arbitrary level. Batchelor and his colleagues (1961) however reported studies of burned children treated by transfusion of plasma without added saline. Their results indicated that the volume of fluid lost increases with increasing size of burn, certainly with burns of up to 60 per cent surface area. Above 60 per cent the rate of increase tends to fall off slightly, but this is of no clinical significance if the transfusion is controlled by careful clinical observation. We conclude therefore that, using the formula and the criteria for control described, there is no need to set any arbitrary upper limit to the volume of transfusion.

The fluids discussed so far have been entirely replacement fluids to make good the loss of constituents of the blood. During the transfusion period the patient will also need an intake of water for ordinary metabolic purposes. Because of the strong antidiuretic factors at work there is reason for believing that the volume of fluid which the kidney can excrete is limited, and that during the first 24-hour period the water intake should be restricted. It is therefore advised that an adult patient should receive only 100 ml of water hourly. If the patient does not vomit then this can be given by mouth in the usual way, and on the second and subsequent days the amount can gradually be increased. If, however, the patient vomits then this metabolic fluid must be added to the drip in the form of glucose in water.

It is easy to give too much water particularly to children and water intoxication has been recorded after drinking quantities which under normal circumstances would have been quite safe.

All deep burns are associated with some loss of red cells and, although the loss of these cells over the shock period is not strictly proportional to the size of the burn, nevertheless the patients with the larger burns do tend to lose more red cells. All patients with deep burns of 10 per cent or more of the body surface should therefore have transfusion of whole blood, and it is advised that a volume of bank blood equivalent to 1 per cent of the patient's blood volume be given for each 1 per cent of surface area involved in deep burning, i.e. an adult patient will require one bottle for each 10 per cent deep burn (Muir, 1961). Some patients may lose blood in larger quantities, and this will be discussed later. It should be pointed out that if blood is given in quantities larger than necessary there is evidence to suggest that it is destroyed more rapidly than normal, and is therefore of no value.

Estimation of the surface area

The rule of nine as advised by Wallace (1951) is recommended for this purpose. This does not give as accurate an estimation of the area involved as other formulae, but it is accurate enough for most practical purposes and is easy to remember (*Figure 2.4*).

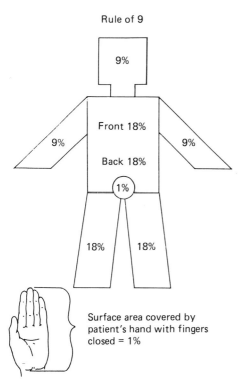

Rule of 9

9%

9%   Front 18%   9%

Back 18%

1%

18%   18%

Surface area covered by patient's hand with fingers closed = 1%

Figure 2.4 Estimation of surface area

For smaller areas a good guide is that the area covered by the patient's hand and fingers is 1 per cent of the body surface. It should be remembered that in children the head is a relatively larger proportion and the lower limbs a relatively smaller proportion of the total body area than in adults. *Figure 2.5* shows the modification necessary for different ages.

Normal measurements

In treating burned patients it is frequently necessary to know such data as weight, blood volume and haematocrit for various ages and sizes, and a table of normal measurements must be available. The one in use in our departments is shown in *Table 2.1*.

CHART FOR ESTIMATING SEVERITY OF BURN WOUND

Name _____ Ward _____ Number _____ Date _____

Age _____   Admission weight_____

Lund and Browder charts

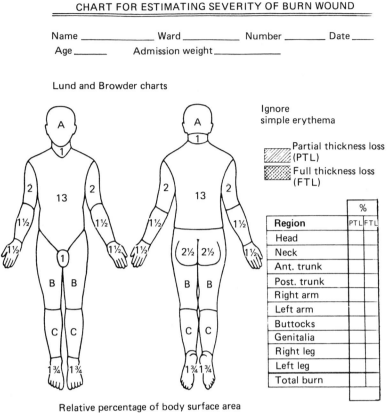

Ignore
simple erythema

Partial thickness loss
(PTL)

Full thickness loss
(FTL)

Region	%	
	PTL	FTL
Head		
Neck		
Ant. trunk		
Post. trunk		
Right arm		
Left arm		
Buttocks		
Genitalia		
Right leg		
Left leg		
Total burn		

Relative percentage of body surface area
affected by growth

Area	Age 0	1	5	10	15	Adult
A = ½ of head	9½	8½	6½	5½	4½	3½
B = ½ of one thigh	2¾	3¼	4	4½	4½	4¾
C = ½ of one leg	2½	2½	2¾	3	3¼	3½

Figure 2.5 Lund and Browder chart for accurate assessment of percentage body surface areas

The practical management of burns shock

(1) Immediately on admission an estimate is made of the total percentage area burned; this includes all the burn except simple erythema.

An estimate is made of the area of full thickness (deep) burning.

If the total percentage area is involved is found to be 15 per cent or more in an adult, or 10 per cent or more in a child, the decision is taken to set up a transfusion with plasma *at once*. Some children with burns of 5–10 per cent of the body surface need transfusion and should be watched carefully.

Site for the drip. Many different types of cannulae and introducers are now available. If a cannula can be easily introduced into a vein by needle puncture, this is done. If, however, no obvious vein is available, a cut-down procedure must be performed without waste of time. This is particularly important in children with extensive burns. Because of venous spasm, drips run badly in

Table 2.1 Table of expected values

Age	Weight (kg) M	F	Height (cm) M	F	Haematocrit M	F	Haemoglobin (%) M	F	Blood vol. (ml) M	F	Metabolic water req. in 1st 24 h (ml/h)	Minimum hourly urine vol. in 1st 24 h
Birth	3.5		50		60		145		260		30	10
6/12	7		65		36		80		520		30	11
1	10		75		38		85		750		30	12
2	12.5		87		38		85		940		30	13
3	15		95		38		85		1120		35	14
4	17		103		39		88		1270		35	15
5	19		110		39		88		1420		40	16
6	22		116		40		90		1650		45	17
7	24		124		40		90		1800		50	18
8	26		130		40		90		1950		55	20
9	30		135		40		90		2250		55	22
10	32		140		40		90		2400		60	24
11	35		145		41	40	93	90	2620		65	26
12	40		150		42	40	96	90	3000		70	29
13	45		156		43	40	98	90	3370		75	32
14	50		160		44	40	100	90	3750		80	35
15	54	52	168	161	44	40	100	90	4050	3800	85	35
16	58	53	172	162	44	40	100	90	4350	4000	90	35
17	62	54	174	163	44	40	100	90	4650	4050	95	35
18	64	55	175	163	44	40	100	90	4800	4120	95	35
Adult	70	60	175	163	44	40	100	90	5000	4500	100	35

legs, and the following are the sites in order of preference: forearm, upper arm, external jugular, leg. If no vein is visible or palpable, a satisfactory vein can always be found by cutting down on the radial border of the forearm at the junction of its lower and middle thirds with the arm in mid-pronation. It is much better to cut down at this site than to insert a catheter at the bend of the elbow. The catheter is introduced for 3 or 4 cm into the vein. We do not advise, except in special circumstances, that polythene catheters should be passed into either of the venae cavae because, in all burns, drip wounds are liable to become infected, and this on occasion has led to septic thrombus formation. If possible the cut-down should be through an area of intact skin, but in extensive burns this is sometimes a counsel of perfection, and under these circumstances it is reasonable to cut down through burned skin and insert the cannula.

Particularly in children there should be no hesitation in using the external jugular vein if necessary, and it will be found that large volumes of fluid can be put in rapidly through this channel. Particular care should be taken to see that the instruments in the cut-down set are suitably fine, because the insertion of a cannula into the collapsed veins of a small child can be an extremely difficult and delicate undertaking.

(2) The weight in kilograms is estimated from:

    (i) Known weight, or ⎫
    (ii) Known height, or ⎬ *see Table 2.1*
    (iii) Age. ⎭

(3) The volume of plasma to be transfused during the *first four hours after injury* is now worked out by the formula:

$$\frac{(\text{Total percentage area of burn} \times \text{weight in kg})}{2} = \text{ml of fluid required.}$$

It must be stressed that this volume should be given in the first four hours after the injury, and not in the first four hours after setting up the transfusion. In practice it will be found that the transfusion is usually started about two hours after burning, and therefore this ration of fluid will be given in two hours.

(4) At the end of the first four-hour period, when the estimated volume of fluid has been given, the patient is examined and particular attention is paid to the following features:

(i)   Restlessness.
(ii) Colour.
(iii) Blood pressure, if distribution of the burn makes it possible to take readings without difficulty.
(iv) Hourly urine volume. Urine to be tested for blood, albumin, sugar and specific gravity.
(v)   Nausea, vomiting or gastric aspirate.
(vi) Haemoglobin or haematocrit level of capillary (e.g. fingerprick) blood.

No single one of the above observations can be relied upon alone to indicate if the transfusion is adequate or not, because under certain circumstances each one of them may give a misleading impression or be difficult of interpretation, and it is necessary by a consideration of all the available facts to determine whether oligaemia has been corrected and the transfusion is keeping pace with the rate of loss, so that the patient remains in a state of compensation. There is no laboratory estimation which will give the surgeon all the information which he requires, and there is no problem which calls for a greater exercise of clinical judgment than assessing the burns patient's condition.

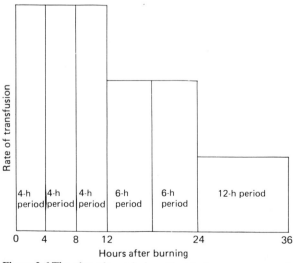

Figure 2.6 The plan of transfusion. The blocks represent equal volumes of fluid

(5) **Progress.** The transfusion is normally carried on until 36 hours after burning, and the time is broken up into six periods as follows (*Figure 2.6*):

1st period	4 hours (from time of burn)
2nd period	4 hours
3rd period	4 hours
4th period	6 hours
5th period	6 hours
6th period	12 hours.

If at the end of the first period the patient's condition is satisfactory then the same volume of plasma (i.e. (wt in kg × percentage area burn)/2 in ml) is given in the subsequent 4-hour period. At the end of the second period the same observations are made as at the end of the first 4-hour period, and if the progress is again satisfactory the plasma ration is continued unchanged to the end of the next period, and so on until six equal volumes of plasma have been given in each of the six periods.* If, however, the clinical condition at the end of a period is unsatisfactory, the plasma ration for the next and subsequent periods must be changed accordingly.

Amounts calculated by this formula are only rarely excessive, and the change most often needed is an increase of the volume because of persistent oligaemia. If it becomes necessary to increase the volume, how can the additional requirement be estimated? Some workers attempt to calculate the plasma volume deficit from the haematocrit, assuming that the red cell volume remains normal, but we believe that this calculation involves so many inaccuracies as to be valueless. A deficit of less than 200 ml (in an adult patient) is not significant, whereas it is unlikely that the deficit in a patient who has been transfused according to the formula will exceed 800 ml. If, therefore, the assessment at the end of a period indicates that the patient is still oligaemic, the plasma 'ration' for the subsequent period should be increased by 200–800 ml according to the clinical condition. Children will require correspondingly smaller increases according to their size.

Particular attention should be paid to the assessment at the end of the first (4-hour) period, and the second (4-hour) period. Because the drip is usually started about two hours after the burn it will be seen that the end of the first 4-hour period will occur when the drip has been running for about two hours, and it is unusual to be able to make an assessment before this time. Occasionally, however, in very extensive burns assessments at these times may be too infrequent, and it may be necessary to examine the patient at the end of each hour. If the volumes are adjusted satisfactorily up to the end of 12 hours, then it is unusual to have to make a great deal of change during the following periods. With the majority of moderately serious burns the transfusion can be safely stopped at 36 hours, if by this time the patient is able to take adequate fluids by mouth. With more extensive burns it may be necessary to continue the transfusion at a slightly diminishing rate to 48 hours or even into the third day.

(6) **Metabolic fluid** requirements must also be met. A start is made by giving 60 ml of water hourly by mouth. If there is no nausea or vomiting this is increased to

---

* The volume of plasma transfused in the first 24 hours is wt in kg × percentage area burn × 2.5 ml. Compare this with the volume given by Evans' formula which is wt in kg × percentage burn × 2.0 ml of which half is plasma and half is normal saline.

100 ml/h (proportionately smaller volumes are given to children – *see Table 2.1*). If nausea or vomiting persists, the metabolic requirements are added to the transfusion in the form of 5 per cent glucose in water. In patients in whom nausea or vomiting persists, and in all patients with burns of over 35 per cent total area, a Ryle's tube is passed and aspiration is performed each hour before fluid is given.

(7) **Catheter.** In all burns of over 25 per cent total area an indwelling urethral catheter is inserted and retained until the transfusion is finished; the urine volume is measured every hour.

A useful rule (Settle, 1974) is that the urine volume should be in the range 0.5–1.0 ml/kg body weight per hour. (*See Table 2.1* for further details.)

(8) **Morphine** is given either intravenously, or into the drip when this has been set up. Great care should be taken if morphine has previously been administered subcutaneously, as this may not be absorbed until the transfusion improves the peripheral circulation, and if a second dose of morphine is given because the first has not worked, then a large quantity of morphine may suddenly be swept into the blood stream and cause serious depression of the patient's respiration.

The dose is 0.2 mg/kg body weight. If papaverine (Omnopon) is preferred, the dose is 0.4 mg/kg body weight.

(9) **Blood.** As soon as convenient a sample of venous blood is withdrawn for determination of blood group, and the serum retained for cross-matching. All patients with deep burns of 10 per cent or more of the surface area need blood transfusion. For each 1 per cent area of deep burn a volume of bank blood equivalent to 1 per cent of the patient's blood volume* is administered. This is given to replace an equivalent volume of plasma as follows:

10–25 per cent area deep burn – during the sixth period.
26–50 per cent area deep burn – partly during the second and
partly during the sixth period.

(10) **Central venous pressure measurement.** If progress is unsatisfactory and particularly if serious impairment of renal function is suspected (*see* p. 44), a central venous catheter should be inserted. If the neck skin is unburned, the catheter should be introduced percutaneously into the internal jugular vein and advanced into the right atrium.

The catheter is introduced as follows (Latimer, 1971): The patient is tipped head down and the head turned towards the opposite side. After injection of local anaesthetic, the skin is punctured at the lateral border of the sternomastoid 3 cm above the clavicle (in an adult). The needle is aimed at the suprasternal notch and advanced deep to the sternomastoid until the vein is entered. The catheter is threaded through the needle and the tip is advanced into the right atrium. The needle is now withdrawn. The catheter is fixed to the skin and connected by a two-way tap to a drip and to the manometer. The insertion of the catheter must be carried out with strict aseptic precautions and the entry wound must be protected by an antiseptic dressing which is changed daily. If the neck is burned the catheter may be inserted through the subclavian vein from below the clavicle (Hardaway, 1968). If neither of these sites is available, a long catheter may be threaded up through a limb vein. The

---

* Total blood volume in ml = wt in kg × 75.

pressure should be measured from the mid-axillary line with the patient in the horizontal position. A safe CVP is in the region of 5–8 cm water. The pressure should not exceed 15 cm.

(11) Temperature measurement. If thermistor probes and a recording instrument are available, a skin probe should be taped to the big toe to record surface temperature and either a rectal probe or an ear probe used to record deep body temperature.

The rectal temperature is normally in the range of 38–40 °C and, under the average warm conditions of an intensive care room, the toe temperature in a patient with no circulatory defect will be 1–4 °C lower. In a patient with uncompensated shock the temperature difference may be as much as 15 °C lower due to compensatory vasoconstriction. The gradual return of this figure to within the normal range is valuable confirmatory evidence of the improvement of the circulation. The rectal or ear probe will also give evidence of the occasional occurrence of hyperpyrexia.

(12) Repeated clinical assessment. It should be repeated that the formula is not stated as a dogma to be followed blindly. It is only used as a general plan for starting the transfusion, and the greatest attention must be paid to the repeated clinical control.

It is often possible to predict, from the circumstances of burning and from the appearance of the burn, if the patient's requirements are liable to deviate markedly from the formula one way or the other. Thus, for instance, the largest loss of fluid is likely to occur in deep partial thickness burns sustained at relatively low temperatures, and with long exposure to the heat, whereas a dry deep burn, in which the skin appears well tanned, may be associated with very much less fluid loss than average. There is also a fairly considerable difference in accordance with the region of the body involved, and in this aspect burns of the face and head are notorious for the large amounts of fluid which may be lost into the relatively lax tissues of the face and neck.

Charting of instructions

The management of the patient will be, for the greater part of the time, in the care of the nursing staff, and it is essential that the clearest instructions should be given if the prescribed treatment is to be carried out correctly.

The type of instruction chart used at Mount Vernon Hospital, is shown in *Figure 2.7.*

Other colloids

Due to the expense and difficulty in obtaining human plasma many attempts have been made to find a satisfactory substitute: gum saline, polyvinylpyrrolidone, dextran and gelatin have all been used; of these only dextran has gained wide acceptance, although the newer gelatin preparation, Haemacell, appears to be of value.

Dextran is a polysaccharide which is produced by polymerization when an organism *Leuconostoc mesenteroides* is grown in a medium of sugar. Dextran can be extracted in a pure state and sterilized. As originally produced, dextran contains molecules of a very wide range of size. It has been found that molecules smaller

BURN SHOCK TREATMENT

Name ....   Weight ....

Time of burn ....   Height ....

Drip up at ....   Total percentage burn area ....

Hb or HTC on admission ....   Percentage area deep burn ....

Formula per period — ...... ✕ ...... ✕ ...... =

First period is from ....to..........		Hb or HTC	Time
Give by drip	Give by drip		
Second period is from .... to		Hb or HTC	Time
Give by mouth	Give by mouth		
Third period is from ....to..........		Hb or HTC	Time
Give by drip	Give by mouth		

Figure 2.7 The chart used for recording instructions of transfusion

than 40 000 molecular weight are rapidly excreted in the urine, whereas molecules larter than 250 000 molecular weight may be harmful.

By suitable extraction methods, it is possible to exclude most of the molecules above and below these limits and the preparations available for clinical use have 80 per cent of the molecules within the molecular weight range 40 000–225 000 (compare the size of the plasma proteins, albumin 69 000, globulin 156 000 and fibrinogen 400 000).

The commercial preparations available consist of fractions between these limits in a 6 per cent solution in normal saline.

The preparations available are as follows:

	Average molecular weight	Proprietary name
Dextran 40	40 000	Rheomacrodex
Dextran 70	70 000	Macrodex, Dextraven 70
Dextran 110	110 000	Intradex (Glaxo), Dextraven 110
Dextran 125	125 000	Dextraven 125
High-molecular-weight dextran	150 000	

Dextran 110 is the preparation most often used in this country and seems to be osmotically closest to human plasma. Dextran 70 has been extensively used in Sweden and in the USA. Dextran 110 has been used by Evans at Roehampton (Evans, 1957, 1969). His programme of administration, the method of control and the total volumes infused are similar to those which we have described for the transfusion of plasma by the Mount Vernon formula. The volumes of Dextran 70 transfused by Sørensen and his colleagues (1967) are also similar to the volumes of plasma which would have been given in similar cases using the Mount Vernon formula. The molecules of dextran are chemically inert and act as substitutes for the lost protein molecules, specifically for the osmotic effect, but they can carry out none of the other functions of the plasma proteins, e.g. transport of antibodies. As plasma loss continues and more dextran is given the proportion of dextran in the blood will rise and the proportion of plasma proteins will fall often to very low levels. This is clearly a theoretical disadvantage. Is it a practical disadvantage? Bull and Jackson (1955) compared two parallel series of cases treated by plasma and by dextran and concluded that the mortality in the dextran series was higher than in the plasma series although only slightly so. A similar attempt was made at Mount Vernon to compare two series of cases treated by plasma and by Dextran 70. The mortality during the shock period in the dextran series was higher than in the plasma series but the causes of some of the deaths were not clear and the result of the trial was inconclusive. It should be noted that in most traumatic conditions and in postoperative cases the volume of dextran which can be given is limited by the tendency of dextran to interfere with clotting mechanisms and it is unusual for more than one plasma volume of dextran to be given over a short period. If dextran is to be used in burns much greater volumes have to be used and, as has been mentioned, Evans and Sørensen have given amounts comparable to the volumes of plasma we use, and which are not uncommonly of the order of 6 litres or more in two days. Clearly, the administration of such volumes is compatible with good recovery.

Treatment by electrolyte solution

The method of transfusion which has been described aims as far as possible to replace like by like, and to keep the body functions close to their normal limits, thus bringing all patients through the shock period with as great a margin of safety as possible. The compensating powers of the body are so great that, particularly in healthy young people, this method of transfusion will result in some patients receiving more fluid than is strictly necessary. For the same reason, it will be obvious that many, indeed probably a majority of patients, can be brought through the shock period by widely differing methods, and by methods which pay much less attention to precise replacement of fluid and maintenance of blood volume. It should, however, be pointed out that simple survival through the shock period is not necessarily an indication of correct or adequate transfusion; the surgeon's aim should be not only to bring the patient through the shock period with as wide a margin of safety as possible, but also to bring him to the end of the shock period in as fit a condition as possible to face the difficulties and dangers of the following weeks. For this reason we feel that no effort should be spared to control the transfusion with accuracy.

Moyer's (1953) cases showed that there was considerable oligaemia in spite of apparently adequate recovery. Moyer concludes from this that oligaemia is not the only factor in the causation of burns shock, and may not even be the most important. His results certainly show that recovery can take place in spite of oligaemia but there is no reason to support that this is desirable if it can be avoided.

In one particular set of circumstances, treatment by Ringer–lactate is particularly valuable: this is when a patient is received late with established hypotensive shock, when rapid transfusion of 2–3 litres of Ringer–lactate is an excellent method for initial treatment, even if another method is to be used later.

Shock treatment by means of electrolyte solution only is now well established and widely used and needs to be considered in detail.

Before going on to the details of treatment we need to consider some fundamental differences in physiological functions between patients treated by colloid regimens and by electrolyte regimens.

In the colloid-treated patient, the most worrying problem is the persistence of low urine volumes even when other signs suggest that the oligaemia has been corrected. In the past, these low urine volumes have been accepted as it was considered that, if the oligaemia had been corrected, then the renal blood flow was normal and that, therefore, the kidney should not be at risk. More recent experience, however, has shown that this may not be so and that a low rate of urine flow under these circumstances may itself contribute to damage to the kidney. On the other hand, a high rate of urine flow appears to provide some advantage to the kidney. Furthermore, irrespective of the blood volume, there is evidence that the urine flow may be influenced by the size of the interstitial space. Two different theories have been proposed to explain the influence of the size of the interstitial space on urine flow: De Wardener (1969) has suggested that the brainstem contains a centre which is sensitive to changes in the size of the interstitial space and that when this becomes distended a hormone is secreted (the natriuretic hormone) which decreases sodium absorption in the proximal convoluted tubule and thus increases urine flow. Conversely, when the interstitial space shrinks this hormone release is inhibited and maximum sodium reabsorption takes place thus diminishing urine flow. Morgan (1969) on the other hand, maintains that changes in the interstitial fluid in the kidney itself alter the shape of the cells of the renal tubules and the intercellular spaces and that this is the controlling mechanism.

It has been explained that one of the natural compensatory mechanisms to the initial loss of plasma volume is for fluid to move from the interstitial space to the plasma under the influence of raised protein osmotic pressure and it may be that transfusion by plasma does not reverse this process, thus allowing a diminished interstitial space to persist. Treatment by electrolyte solution alone is invariably associated with a large increase in size of the undamaged part of the interstitial space (as well as that at the site of the the burn) and, whichever of the above theories is correct, this may be beneficial in increasing urine output.

Sørensen and Sejrsen (1965) gave a well-documented account of 32 patients with severe burns who were given only saline as shock treatment. Control of shock was good and the only deaths which occurred during the period were due to lung damage. There were no cases of acute renal failure. The total volumes of fluid administered to these patients were very large and exceeded the volumes worked out by the Mount Vernon formula by a factor of at least two and, in some cases, by a factor of six. Sørensen and Sejrsen particularly commented on extensive generalized oedema. The volumes transfused by Moyer (1965) were smaller than those of Sørensen and Sejrsen.

However, the high haematocrit readings (sometimes up to 60 per cent) and the low CVP readings (0–1 cmH$_2$O) in the electrolyte-treated cases indicate that blood volumes remain low and, in spite of the high urine flows, there must remain anxiety about the effects of the hypovolaemia on other viscera. Muir and Jones (1976) compared the very low incidence of duodenal ulceration (Curling's ulcer) in the UK with that in the USA and suggested that this might be because at that time plasma was used exclusively in the UK as opposed to electrolytes in the USA.

Treatment by electrolyte transfusion

The initial assessment is as described for plasma transfusion and the same time periods can be used.

The fluid is preferably Ringer–lactate (Hartmann's) solution and the volume of solution to be given in the first 4-hour period is obtained from the formula weight (in kg) × percentage area. The urine flow is the most important indication of the adequacy of treatment and the aim should be an hourly urine volume of 50 ml. Even with this or with higher urine flows, the haematocrit remains high indicating that hypovolaemia is not corrected. Similarly CVP readings remain low and cannot be raised to normal even when very large volumes of fluid are given (Masterton and Dudley, 1971).

The volume of transfused fluid may have to be much increased over the suggested formula and, in a single period, may be as much as weight (in kg) × percentage area burn × ⅚ ml.

Other electrolyte regimens

The electrolyte solutions which have been described so far have all been isotonic with electrolyte concentrations similar to those in normal plasma. However the large volumes which it is necessary to give have often caused excessive enlargement of the extracellular space. This has sometimes caused gross oedema of unburned parts of the body and has also been blamed as at least one of the causes of shock lung.

For this reason and by concentrating exclusively on the deficit of sodium to the exclusion of other factors, Monafo (1970) has suggested that treatment should be by means of a hypertonic solution of sodium chloride and lactate. This exclusion of other factors seems illogical and the method has not been widely adopted.

Treatment by predetermined volumes of electrolytes

The regimens which have been described so far depend upon frequent observation and continuous control of the transfusion but circumstances may arise when for one reason or another this type of supervision is impossible. Under these circumstances, patients can benefit from transfusion of a predetermined volume of Ringer–lactate solution as follows:

Adults receive a volume of solution equivalent to 10 per cent of body weight during the first 24 hours and 5 per cent of body weight during the second 24 hours.

Children receive a volume equivalent to 11 per cent of body weight in the first 24 hours and 6 per cent of body weight in the second 24 hours.

Even if it were not possible to give fluid intravenously, a situation which might occur in a mass disaster, similar volumes of fluid could be given to those patients who were able to drink without vomiting. For this purpose Markley and his colleagues (1956) suggested the following solution:

Sodium chloride	– 5.5 g	This gives	Sodium	140 mequiv./l
Sodium bicarbonate	– 4.0 g	a solution	Chloride	93 mequiv./l
Water	– 1 l	containing	Bicarbonate	47 mequiv./l

Mixed electrolyte and plasma regimens

In the light of the discussion on previous pages it might seem that a mixed plasma and electrolyte regimen should be able to combine the advantages of the two systems, i.e. maintenance of good blood volume and satisfactory urine flow. As has been mentioned, transfusion by various mixtures of plasma and electrolytes were much used in the past although the reasons for their use were often different from those expounded above.

An example of a combined colloid–electrolyte transfusion is that of Stone and his colleagues (1969) who advise using an electrolyte (saline and bicarbonate) and plasma mixture in the proportion of 3 to 1.

More recently a saline–plasma combination has been used in a different way. Baxter (1971) has suggested that only electrolytes should be given in the first 24 hours since during this time the protein molecules of transfused plasma are lost, at the site of the burn, as rapidly as the electrolyte molecules and therefore convey no benefit. However, by the second day the damaged capillaries will be recovering, protein molecules will be retained in the circulation and therefore plasma can be given with benefit at that time. The difference in haematocrits in the first 24 hours between cases treated with either plasma or electrolytes make it difficult to accept the hypothetical basis of this treatment but it remains as a possible improvement on an electrolyte only regimen.

Treatment of patients not requiring transfusion

In this category are burns of less than 15 per cent surface area in adults or 10 per cent in children. These patients do not tend to vomit and they can be managed successfully by the oral administration of fluids. Unless the burn is trivial, intake and output measurements should be made and charted, and in those patients with burns close to the critical levels, clinical assessment should be made at suitable intervals to ensure that progress is satisfactory. Patients with burns of the face should be observed particularly, for they tend to lose fluid out of proportion to the size of the area involved.

Hypotonic solutions are tolerated better than isotonic solution, when given by mouth, and are preferred for this group of patients, although for more extensive burns most workers have advised isotonic solution (*see* p. 33).

A suitable hypotonic solution can be made by dissolving 3 g salt and 1.5 g sodium bicarbonate in one litre of water (half a teaspoon of salt and half a teaspoon of sodium bicarbonate in 2 pints of water). This can be flavoured with orange squash.

Volumes can be calculated over longer periods than the volumes for intravenous infusions and a simple rule is to give (wt in kg × total percentage area burn × 4) ml in the first 12 hours after the burn and the same volume again in the next 24 hours.

Oxygen
Some authorities have advised the use of oxygen because shocked patients may be blue. The blueness, however, is due to poor circulation in the capillaries and will be

relieved by adequate transfusion. Oxygen need be given only if respiratory damage has occurred.

Toxins
In order to explain certain features of the clinical course of burns shock, it has been postulated at various times that toxic substances are produced as a result of damage to the tissues by heat, and that these are absorbed by the blood stream, producing deleterious effects (Wilson, MacGregor and Stewart, 1938). Histamine, adenosine compounds, polypeptides and abnormal proteins have all been implicated at one time or another. It is true that all these compounds can be produced by the effect of heat on tissues, and that they can cause serious illness if injected into experimental animals. On the other hand, no direct evidence is available that they are responsible for shock in man, and most of the effects for which they have been blamed have gradually been explained by increasing knowledge of circulatory dynamics and other factors.

The manifestations of what used to be called acute toxaemia were the manifestations of oligaemia, and do not occur with adequate transfusion.

It is interesting to note that the early liver necrosis, which, in the 1930s, was thought to be due to toxaemia, was found to be due to absorption of tannic acid which, at that time, was in favour as a local application.

Other toxic effects were undoubtedly due to severe early sepsis. Fortunately sepsis during the shock period is now rare.

Other aspects of the effects of toxins are discussed later.

Antihistamines
In the light of the theory that the capillary dilatation and increased permeability are due to locally released histamine, attempts have been made to influence the loss of fluid by the use of antihistamines. A number of enthusiastic and uncritical reports have advocated this treatment, but none of these claims has been borne out by a controlled clinical trial or by experimental observation, and we believe that there is no indication for the use of these drugs in the treatment of burns shock (Butterfield, 1957; Sevitt, 1957).

Cortisone and ACTH
These drugs have also been used in burned patients in attempts to influence the permeability of the damaged capillaries, and also for less clearly specified reasons. There is no evidence that adrenocortical activity is deficient in burns shock, or that administration of these hormones has any beneficial effects, and therefore they should not be given (Butterfield, 1957; Sevitt, 1957).

Calcium
Calcium has also been administered in order to reduce capillary permeability and limit fluid loss. However, there is no evidence that it has any effect in this direction. Recently suggestions have been made that a fall in ionizable calcium may occur because of the quantity of citrate absorbed during a rapid plasma transfusion, and two workers have reported deterioration of clinical condition relieved by injection of calcium gluconate (H. Gemmeke, 1960, personal communication; J. Kirk, 1960, personal communication). Unfortunately, estimation of ionizable calcium is exceptionally difficult, and it has not so far been possible to follow this work any further.

Cold water treatment (*see* Chapter 7)
The treatment of burns by immersion in cold water has been practised for many years and, indeed, reflection makes one feel that it may have been a method of treatment even in prehistoric days. Anyone who has used it on himself for a minor painful burn will have no doubt of the symptomatic relief which it affords, but at the moment it seems unlikely that it can be used to influence the course of shock in an extensive burn.

Complications during the shock period

Some of the complications which are discussed here actually become manifest after the shock phase, but they either have their origin during that period or form part of the complex metabolic disturbances which follow directly from these, so that we have thought it more convenient to group them together.

Disturbances of electrolytes

During the discussion of replacement transfusion by plasma, the argument has been pursued as though all the solutions involved were of equivalent electrolyte concentration, and the balance of electrolytes has largely been ignored. Although some disturbances of the electrolyte pattern do exist, nevertheless it is right that the emphasis during the first few days should be firmly on the problem of maintenance of volume, because if the blood volume can be satisfactorily maintained so that by the second day the patient is able to take by mouth good quantities of mixed fluids, and if the kidneys are able to function satisfactorily, the electrolyte pattern will gradually return to normal. Harmful electrolyte disturbances are infrequent, but if they do occur management may be very difficult, for not only is there a loss of electrolytes from the surface of the burn which is impossible to measure except under difficult experimental conditions, but also the oedema fluid at the site of the burn, being in constant exchange with the fluid and electrolytes of the blood, provides a huge reservoir, the size and behaviour of which is extremely difficult to predict. Reliance must be placed on serial estimations of blood electrolyte levels and also on the estimation of total electrolytes in 24-hour urine specimens. With this information it may be possible, by adjusting the intake of the different electrolytes, to expedite a return to normal levels.

In dealing with electrolyte disturbances, it is usual to assume that the properties of the cell membranes remain constant, i.e. that the cells are perfect osmometers, and that the concentrations of substances in the extracellular fluid have a fixed relationship to the concentrations in the intracellular fluid. There is now evidence that, in a small proportion of burned patients, the cell membranes may become abnormal, allowing potassium to leak out and sodium to enter in an abnormal amount, so that it is no longer possible to predict the levels of intracellular electrolyte from measurement of electrolytes in the blood plasma. Indeed, the blood plasma measurements may be within normal limits in the presence of severe intracellular changes. This condition has been called the 'sick-cell syndrome' (Allison, Hinton and Chamberlain, 1968; Flear *et al.*, 1969; Hinton and Allison, 1969).

In burned patients, this occurs late during the shock period or even after the shock period has ended and results in a characteristic clinical picture of which the features are restlessness, disorientation and overbreathing. No reliance can be placed on the electrolyte levels in the blood plasma, but a clue may be gained from examination of 24-hour urine specimens, which show a reversal of the usual sodium to potassium ratio (normally approximately 2:1). The first step in treatment is to make sure that no correctable cause of tissue hypoxia is still present. The most likely cause at this stage is the presence of an unrecognized deficit of red cells. This should be corrected by blood transfusion. The administration of insulin and glucose also has a beneficial effect in restoring the cell membranes to normal, and Hinton and Allison (1969) have suggested that 150–200 units of insulin and 1–2 litres of 5 per cent glucose should be given daily.

Massive red cell destruction

Some account has already been given of the usual pattern of red cell destruction in severe burns. In the first few hours the amount of red cell destruction bears a relationship to the size of the burn, although even in deep burns of up to 50 per cent body surface, loss of more than 10 per cent of the red cell volume is rare. Early haemoglobinuria is common in patients with severe burns, but usually clears rapidly over the first few hours. Red cell fragility curves of the blood in these patients shows a marked tail of abnormally fragile cells and a shift of the body of the curve to the right. As the haemoglobinaemia fades the tail of the curve disappears and the curve as a whole moves to the left (*Figure 2.8a*).

Patients whose curves follow this pattern lose only moderate amounts of red cells, as has already been discussed.

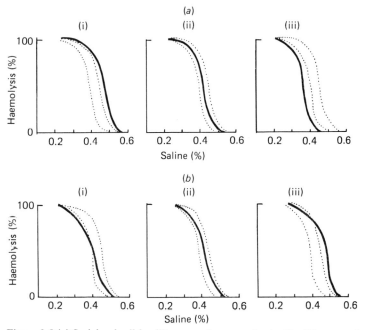

Figure 2.8 (*a*) Serial red cell fragility curves from a patient with a 30 per cent burn. The curves move progressively to the left. This patient destroyed only a moderate number of red cells. (*b*) Serial fragility curves from another patient with a 40 per cent burn. The curves move progressively to the right. This patient destroyed a large volume of red cells. Neither of these patients showed a 'tail' (cf. *Figure 2.1*)

Some patients, however, show a rapidly increasing rate of loss, and a volume of red cells equivalent to the original red cell volume may be destroyed (Muir, 1961). The fragility curves of these patients may move progressively to the right (*Figure 2.8b*).

Signs which should raise suspicion of massive red cell destruction are:

(i) Failure of the patient to respond to treatment even when the haematocrit is falling.

(ii) Haemoglobinuria occurring for the first time 12 hours or more after burning when the urine has previously been clear or, alternatively, recurring after complete or partial clearance of an early haemoglobinuria.

Under these circumstances serial red cell fragility estimations should be done, and the surgeon should be prepared to transfuse large volumes of blood, as great as or greater than the patient's estimated normal blood volume.

Renal failure

It is evident that renal failure is a potential complication in any patient with a large burn. Unless resuscitation with appropriate intravenous fluids is started early and continued effectively, the inevitable fall in cardiac output can be sufficient to reduce the effective renal perfusion to the point where classical acute tubular necrosis occurs. In the vast majority of burn patients, effective intravenous fluid therapy will prevent this very serious complication. However, if effective treatment is delayed, renal failure can occur even in patients with relatively small burns. For example, a 60-year-old previously healthy male was admitted to the Yorkshire Regional Burns Centre 12 hours after he had sustained a deep flame burn to his right buttock, thigh and leg amounting to 10 per cent of his body surface area. He had not sought any medical assistance until 10 hours post-burn and, within a few hours of admission to the Burns Centre, it was evident that oliguric renal failure was established. So catabolic was this patient that his blood urea level rose at a rate of over 15 mmol/24 hour until checked by peritoneal dialysis. Subsequently, repeated haemodialysis was required to control his uraemia. At three weeks, spontaneous recovery of renal function commenced and, after the burn wounds had been closed by skin grafting, he was discharged home with perfectly satisfactory renal function 13 weeks after the injury.

Occasionally, patients with extensive burns develop early renal failure in spite of apparently adequate fluid therapy. For example, a 10-year-old boy with 55 per cent mainly very deep burns was admitted to the Yorkshire Regional Burns Centre during the third hour post-burn, effective intravenous fluid therapy having been commenced during the previous hour. In spite of rapid correction of moderate haemoconcentration, his urine output remained inadequate (mean value 0.5 ml/h per kg but with osmolarity fixed at about 350 mosmol/l). Peritoneal dialysis was commenced at 54 hours post-burn (blood urea 34 mmol/l; potassium 6.2 mmol/l) and was continued for 10 days. Three major skin grafting sessions were required and he was discharged home 18 weeks after the injury. (Details of this case have previously been published – Settle, 1974.)

The gravity of renal failure as a complication of burns can hardly be overstated. Because the survival of the patient during the first 36 hours following extensive burns is dependent upon the infusion of vast quantities of fluid, it is inevitable that by the second and third days post-burn there will be a large positive fluid balance in the form of burn oedema. Resolution of this burn oedema occurs as a consequence of a reverse shift from interstitial to intravascular compartments followed by diuresis. If this diuresis is not possible, and it certainly is not if renal failure supervenes, the burn oedema will be redistributed to the lungs and severe pulmonary oedema will occur. The extensively burned patient, whose kidneys fail during or soon after effective fluid resuscitation, is likely to drown in his own extracellular fluid long before hyperkalaemia reaches a fatal level; hence the need for early diagnosis and urgent and effective treatment of renal failure following extensive burns.

Diagnosis of renal impairment
It is our experience that all patients with burns of more than 20 per cent show some evidence of mixed glomerular and tubular damage during the first few days post-burn (Yu *et al.*, 1983). This damage shows itself in the form of proteinuria comprising high-molecular-weight proteins such as albumin (mol. wt 66 300), low-molecular-weight proteins such as β_2-microglobulin (mol. wt 11 800) and tubular enzymes such as *N*-acetyl-β-D-glucosaminidase (NAG). The severity of total proteinuria is directly related to the severity of the burn, but this phase of mixed glomerular and tubular proteinuria usually resolves once the patient is stabilized by effective resuscitation. There then follows a period of tubular proteinuria characterized by increased excretion of low-molecular-weight proteins and a rising level of NAG. The final return to normal proximal tubular cell function in an uncomplicated patient may take several weeks. The initial proteinuria may be accompanied by other indications of acute renal insufficiency, such as a falling glomerular filtration rate and failure to concentrate the urine, but if these are absent, renal damage is insufficient to affect normal excretory function of the kidney and its role in maintaining body water and electrolyte balance. However, these studies, together with routine urine osmometry during the last 17 years, have demonstrated a spectrum of renal impairment ranging from a transient and relatively insignificant proteinuria through to acute oliguric renal failure with total loss of urine-concentrating power characteristic of acute tubular necrosis.

Acute oliguric renal failure occurring early in the shock phase should be diagnosed within hours of its onset. The characteristic findings are: (*a*) very low hourly urine volumes, e.g. 10 ml/h or less in an adult, (*b*) loss of urine concentration/dilution power with a 'fixed' urine osmolarity of about 350 mosmol/l, (*c*) urine:blood urea ratio of 5 or less, (*d*) high Na^+ and low K^+ levels in urine, (*e*) low urine creatinine levels, (*f*) rising blood creatinine level with very low creatinine clearance (10 ml/min or less), (*g*) uraemia – azotaemia, hyperkalaemia, hyponatraemia and metabolic acidosis.

At the other end of the spectrum, there is minor tubular damage in which the maximum urine concentration may be limited to 500 mosmol/l and urine:blood urea ratio lies in the range 15–20. This abnormality will be detected only if it is looked for actively or if urine osmolarity (or urea-concentrating power) measurement is a frequent and routine investigation. If the patient is kept in good fluid and electrolyte balance, this minor impairment of renal function will be of little significance. However, if the patient becomes hypernatraemic and hyperosmolar as a consequence of losing sodium-free water that is not being replaced (most likely if the burn wound is being treated by exposure and the vast evaporative water losses have not been appreciated), the inability of the kidney to correct body osmolar balance by excreting a highly concentrated urine may be a critical factor in the development of progressive hyperosmolarity.

Between these two extremes lies non-oliguric (or high output) renal failure. As Cason pointed out in 1966, when he reported a 5 per cent incidence of renal failure in a series of 962 burn patients who had required active resuscitation, about half the cases of post-burn renal failure are of a non-oliguric type. Ten years previously, Sevitt (1956) had described the postmortem appearance of the kidney in such cases and concluded that the underlying pathology was a necrosis of the distal convoluted tubule, the condition being called 'lower nephron nephrosis'. Commonly, the complication is not recognized in the early stages since urine flow may seem to be adequate, and the unexpected finding of a high blood urea level at the end of the shock phase or even several days later may be the first indication that a serious complication has occurred. This unpleasant surprise can be avoided if the quality of the urine is examined in addition to measuring its quantity. Typically, the urine concentration in non-oliguric failure will lie in the 350–400 mosmol/l range and the urine:blood urea ratio will be less than 10 and may be less than 5 (compare the normal of over 50). Often there will be casts in the urine and, in a high proportion of cases, a history of 'haemoglobinuria' during the early stages of the shock phase.

It may be thought that routine measurement of blood urea would also provide early warning of impending or actual renal failure. In our experience it is less useful than urine osmolarity measurement because many burn patients with good renal function can have a temporary rise in blood urea to levels between 10 and 15 mmol/l simply because of the hypercatabolism that accompanies the burn injury. Furthermore, we have seen blood urea levels of over 30 mmol/l in patients whose renal impairment was relatively minor and who certainly did not require dialysis.

Management of renal impairment
The early recognition of loss of renal-concentrating power is essential for two separate reasons. First, it allows the clinician the option of attempting to restore renal function and, if this fails, to proceed with forms of treatment designed to prevent uraemia. Secondly, it signals the end of urine flow measurement as any sort of index of effective resuscitation. If the burn is extensive and the renal impairment judged to be serious, it is advisable to institute CVP measurement. This will provide a reliable means of judging the fluid therapy requirement in circumstances where the response to overtransfusion will be pulmonary oedema rather than diuresis.

There are occasions when persistent and inappropriate vasoconstriction may be responsible for 'physiological' impairment of renal function. This complication can be avoided if small doses of chlorpromazine are used during the shock phase, for in addition to its sedative and anti-emetic properties, it also has some alpha-receptor blocking activity. A much more powerful drug in this respect is phenoxybenzamine, but it should only be used with great care since its administration may be followed by a catastrophic fall in blood pressure. The doctor should be satisfied by CVP measurement that blood volume replacement has been adequate before phenoxybenzamine is given (0.5 mg/kg body wt, given in 250 ml of 0.9 per cent saline over 30 minutes). CVP monitoring must be continued whilst the drug is being given and it is highly likely that additional fluid will need to be given to fill the vessels released from vasoconstriction.

When the renal impairment is of the non-oliguric type, the possibility of producing a diuresis should be considered. If the urine sodium is less than 10 mmol/l, the tubule may respond to frusemide (1 mg/kg body wt given intravenously). Otherwise, a solute diuretic such as mannitol can be tried (1 g/kg body wt given as a 20 per cent solution over 15–30 minutes). When mannitol works satisfactorily, the response is an obvious diuresis that continues, though gradually declining, over the next 12 hours. If it does not work, it *must not* be repeated as this may lead to sudden pulmonary oedema. If a urine flow of several litres per day can be maintained by the use of a diuretic, urinary excretion of urea, potassium etc. may be sufficient to prevent uraemia. However, very careful attention will need to be paid to the patient's water and electrolyte balance and blood chemistry measurements should be performed at least twice a day.

If a satisfactory diuresis cannot be induced, it is best to proceed to dialysis at an early stage. Because the patient will very probably by hypercatabolic, conservative methods of management are seldom useful. Unless the clinician in charge of the burn patient is experienced in the techniques of dialysis, it will be best to obtain the advice and assistance of a renal physician. However, peritoneal dialysis is a relatively straight-forward technique that can reasonably be undertaken by any clinician who is competent to look after patients with severe burns.

Technique of peritoneal dialysis
This can be performed though burned skin although intact skin is obviously preferred. Dialysis fluid, administration sets, catheters, and collection bags are commercially available, and carry clear instructions. Briefly, the technique is as follows:

(1) Empty the bladder.
(2) Choose the site of insertion (midline, one-third down from the umbilicus to the pubis, is best).
(3) Infiltrate the site with local anaesthetic, and incise the skin with a scalpel.
(4) Push the trochar, with obturator in place, into the peritoneal cavity.
(5) Remove the obturator, and push the trochar in further.
(6) Insert the cannula so that it lies in the left paracolic gutter, and test for patency before securing with a purse-string suture.

The principle of peritoneal dialysis is to run dialysate into the abdominal cavity, allow it to equilibrate with the blood in the mesenteric vessels, syphon it out and then run in some more. For an adult, 2 litres of dialysate would be used and each complete cycle would take about one hour. The whole procedure may need to be continued for up to two weeks and great care must be taken to avoid peritonitis due to bacterial contamination of the fluids or the equipment. Useful instructions and advice come with the commercial dialysate which is available in two main forms. One has a glucose content of 1.36 per cent and is moderately hypertonic whilst the other, with 6.36 per cent glucose, is strongly hypertonic and is used when the removal of a large positive water balance is required.

Haemodialysis
The authors have experience of several patients in whom the combination of acute oliguric renal failure and hypercatabolism due to extensive burns resulted in blood urea levels rising at the rate of 15–20 mmol/l per day. With this rate of urea production it is unlikely that peritoneal dialysis will be able to stop the blood urea level from rising and haemodialysis will be required. In a recent case, haemodialysis using equipment with the maximal clearance rate available, had to be repeated twice a day in order to control the blood urea level. This requirement was unprecedented in the experience of the renal physician concerned.

If gross overhydration is the main problem, the possibility of using a technique of ultrafiltration rather than dialysis should be considered.

'Haemoglobinuria'

Thermally degraded haem pigments from haemoglobin and myoglobin have a sinister reputation for producing renal damage, although the normal kidney can pass large quantities of normal haemoglobin without any damage occurring. Whether the urinary pigments sometimes seen in patients with deep or extensive burns are actually responsible for renal damage, or whether some other 'toxic' substance is responsible, is not yet clear. However, a diuresis that will clear haem pigments will also clear any other 'toxic' substance present and most burn clinicians will give mannitol (1 g/kg body wt given intravenously as a 20 per cent solution over 15–30 min). The caution given above about repeating mannitol should be observed. Most burn clinicians believe, like Dudley, Batchelor and Sutherland (1957), that they have, at some time, aborted renal failure by using mannitol but objective proof is difficult to find.

The prognosis of renal failure

Twenty years ago, post-burn renal failure was considered to be virtually always a fatal event (Cameron and Miller Jones, 1967), and only a handful of survivors had been reported in the world literature. The position today is rather different. Early diagnosis and effective treatment can be expected to give the patient a good chance of surviving this complication. Subsequently, until he is healed, the patient's chance of surviving is probably not much worse than if his burn had not been complicated by renal failure.

Gastric and duodenal ulceration

Superficial gastric erosions are common in the first few days after burning injuries. They are usually multiple and may produce small amounts of blood which is detectable in gastric aspiration.

True duodenal ulceration has been known about for many years and becomes manifest 10–14 days after injury. This is the ulcer which was described by Curling in 1842 and is usually known by his name. This ulcer may bleed or perforate. The incidence of Curling's ulcer in reports from the USA has been shown to be as high as 5 per cent whereas, in the UK, Muir and Jones (1976) could only find 18 definite examples out of approximately 32 500 cases treated in units admitting major burns. Searching for a reason for the marked difference, Muir and Jones pointed out that in the USA cases, shock treatment had been predominantly by electrolyte solutions whereas the UK cases had been treated by plasma. The differences in the physiological status of patients in these two groups which has already been described may explain the difference. Whatever the precise mechanism of causation, it seems likely that the initial damage occurs during the shock period and is a result of unrecognized or uncorrected oligaemia intensified by the defence mechanism of visceral vasoconstrictor.

Shock lung – respiratory distress syndrome

This has been reported more frequently in burned patients in recent years, but whether this represents a true increase in incidence or whether it is being recognized more often is not known. Its high incidence in battle casualties given large volumes of electrolytes suggests that enlargement of the interstitial space in the lungs may be a causative factor.

Other complications

Liver failure, necrosis of the pancreas and necrosis of the gallbladder have also been described after severe burns. The causes are probably similar to those of duodenal ulcers.

Glycosuria and hyperglycaemia
These conditions (Bailey, 1966) require special mention. They may present as:

Transient glycosuria without ketonuria   This is common. When it occurs the first or second specimen of urine contains sugar. The condition lasts up to 48 hours, is unaccompanied by symptoms, and is thought to be due to adrenal medullary over-response to stress. No treatment is required.

Exacerbation of pre-existent diabetes mellitus   This or unmasking of incipient diabetes, evidenced by glycosuria, ketonuria and raised blood sugar levels, will respond to insulin treatment in the usual way.

Pseudodiabetes of burns   This condition, thought to be due to adrenal cortical overaction, is much more serious. It appears several days after burning, well beyond the shock phase, and is characterized by gross glycosuria and hyperglycaemia of up to 1000 mg/100 ml. Ketosis is not a feature. The condition is resistant to insulin even in very large dosage, and lasts for several weeks with slowly diminishing intensity. Two untoward effects are gross wasting due to excessive catabolism and mental disturbance, sometimes even transient psychosis. The treatment recommended for this rare condition is high calorie feeding (*see* p. 99) in an attempt to spare the protein catabolism, and insulin therapy, with the intention of protecting pancreatic islet cells.

Hopeless cases
The facilities available for the treatment of burns shock make it possible for almost all patients, no matter how severe their injuries are, to survive through the shock period. In the present state of our knowledge, however, patients with burns above a critical size invariably succumb after having lived in great pain and misery for a few days or weeks.

The relationship between increasing age and the decreasing size of burn which will be fatal has already been discussed in Chapter 1, and a simplified form of 'probability chart' is reproduced in *Figure 2.9*.

The surgeon will sometimes be faced with the situation where the age of the patient and the size of his burn put him in the category where recovery is unknown. The question must then be asked whether it is not more humane to give only symptomatic treatment and to make the patient as comfortable as possible, while awaiting the inevitable end, than to persevere with resuscitation regardless of the outcome. We believe that this is a proper question for the surgeon to ask himself and that when the indications are clear it is his duty to withhold active resuscitation, but to give as much symptomatic relief as possible.

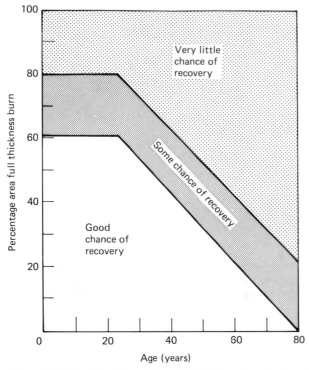

Figure 2.9 A simplified form of 'probability' chart showing how the chances of recovery vary with the size of the burn and the age of the patient. None of our patients whose coordinates met in the darkly stippled part of the graph survived, and for such patients, therefore, the possibility of giving only symptomatic treatment should always be considered

It goes without saying that the decision should be made only by a senior and experienced surgeon and that, if he is not immediately available, the man on the spot should carry out resuscitation on the usual lines pending his arrival.

Since a deep burn is of much more serious import than a superficial one, and to ensure that possible survivors are not abandoned, it is suggested that in making the decision to withhold active treatment, the *area of deep burning only* should be considered. In the authors' units, there has been no recovery of any patient whose coordinates met in the darkly shaded part of the chart, and when such a patient is first seen, the question of giving only symptomatic treatment should always be considered. In making the final decision, factors such as the distribution of the burn, the availability of possible donor sites and the normal expectation of life should be taken into account, as well as the age of the patient and the size of the burn.

Summary of treatment of burns shock

(1) *Estimate* – using 'rule of nine'.
    (i) *Total percentage area burned.* This to include all burn except simple erythema.
    (ii) *Percentage area of full thickness burn* (deep burn).

(2) *Estimate weight* in kg from:
 (i)   Known weight, or
 (ii) measured weight, or
 (iii) age.

(3) *All adults with burns of 15 per cent body surface* or more, and *all children with burns of 10 per cent body surface* or more, need immediate transfusion with plasma. Some children with burns of 5–10 per cent body surface need transfusion and should be watched carefully.

(4) *Set up intravenous drip.* Particularly with children, do not waste time trying to insert a needle. Cut down. Drips run badly in legs and the following are the sites of preference: forearm, upper arm, external jugular, leg.

(5) *Volume of plasma* to be transfused is given by the formula:

$$\frac{\text{Total percentage area of burn} \times \text{weight in kg}}{2} = \text{ml of plasma.}$$

This volume is to be given by 4 hours *from time of the burn* (first period). Four hours from time of burn – the patient's condition is assessed and, if it is satisfactory, the same volume of plasma is given again during the next 4 hours (second period). The patient's condition is again assessed and, if satisfactory, the same volume of plasma is given in the next 4 hours (third period), next 6 hours (fourth period), next 6 hours (fifth period) and next 12 hours (sixth period), an assessment being made at the end of each period.
 This plan therefore involves giving six equal 'rations' of plasma in six periods of varying length and carries the transfusions on to 36 hours after burning.

(6) *Observations to be made at the end of each period:*

 (i)   Presence or absence of restlessness.
 (ii) Colour.
 (iii) Blood pressure.
 (iv) Urine volume.
 (v)   Nausea, vomiting or gastric aspirate.
 (vi) Capillary haemoglobin or haematocrit level.

(7) *Progress and control.* If the assessment at the end of a period shows a satisfactory state, the transfusion is continued as in (5) above. If the patient's condition is not satisfactory, the plasma rations for the next and subsequent periods will be changed.
 Amounts calculated by this formula are only rarely excessive and the change most often needed is an increase in amount because of persistent oligaemia.
 Particular attention should be paid to the assessment at the end of the first (4-hour) and second (4-hour) periods.

(8) *Urine* to be collected and tested hourly. In burns over 35 per cent insert indwelling catheter and retain until transfusion is finished.

(9) If progress is unsatisfactory and urine output causes anxiety, insert a central venous pressure cannula.

(10) *Oral fluids – metabolid fluid requirement.* Water must also be given for metabolic fluid requirements. Start by giving 60 ml of water hourly by mouth for an adult (proportionately less for children). If there is no nausea or vomiting, this may be increased to 100 ml hourly. If nausea or vomiting persist, add the metabolic requirements to the transfusion in the form of 5 per cent glucose and water.

In burns over 35 per cent total area, pass Ryle's tube and aspirate each hour before the fluid is given.

(11) *Morphine* should be given intravenously or into the drip.

(12) *Blood.* Patients with 10 per cent area or more of deep burn should have blood transfusions.

For each 1 per cent area of deep burn give a volume of bank blood equal to 1 per cent of the patient's total blood volume. (Blood volume = weight in kg × 75 ml.) This should be given in place of plasma:

10–25 per cent area deep burn – during sixth period.
26–50 per cent area deep burn – partly during the second and
                                                    partly during the sixth period.

(13) The formula gives only an approximate extimate of expected loss and is intended only as a guide to start with.

It is a help to remember that:

(*a*) Patients with burns over 30 per cent often need the transfusion continued for 48 or 72 hours.
(*b*) Patients with burns of face lose more plasma than those with burns of comparable size in other areas.

(14) *Dextran.* Plasma is considered to be superior to dextran and should be used if available. If dextran is used the management is the same as for plasma.

References

AIKAWA, N., MARTYN, J. A. J. and BURKE, J. F. (1978) Pulmonary artery catheterization and thermodilution cardiac output determination in the management of critically burned patients. *American Journal of Surgery,* **138,** 811

ALLISON, S. P., HINTON, P. and CHAMBERLAIN, M. J. (1968) Intravenous glucose tolerance, insulin and free fatty acid levels in burned patients. *Lancet,* **ii,** 1113

ARTZ, C. P. and REISS, E. (1957) *Treatment of Burns.* Philadelphia: W. B. Saunders Co.

BAILEY, B. N. (1960) Hyperglycaemia in burns. *British Medical Journal,* **2,** 1783

BARTON, G. M. and LAING, J. E. (1970) Control of intravenous therapy by blood volume estimations. In *Transactions of the Third International Congress on Research in Burns.* Prague, 20–25 September 1970. Eds P. Matter, T. L. Barclay and Z. Konickova, pp. 87–90. Berne: Hans Huber

BATCHELOR, A. D. R., KIRK, J. and SUTHERLAND, A. (1961) Treatment of shock in the burned child. *Lancet,* **i,** 123

BAXTER, C. R. (1971) Crystalloid resuscitation of burn shock. In *Contemporary Burn Management.* Eds H. C. Polk and H. H. Stone, pp. 7–32. Boston: Little, Brown

BULL, J. P. and JACKSON, D. McG. (1955) In *Dextran: Its Properties and Use in Medicine.* Oxford: Blackwell Scientific

BUTTERFIELD, W. J. H. (1957) Flash burns from atomic weapons. II. Treatment of shallow blister flash burns by trials of promethazine, adrenaline, cortisone and adrenocorticotrophic hormone. *Surgery, Gynecology and Obstetrics,* **104,** 53

CAMERON, J. S. and MILLER JONES, C. M. (1967) Renal function and renal failure in badly burned children. *British Journal of Surgery,* **54,** 132

CASON, J. S. (1966) Treatment of renal failure. *Transactions of the 2nd International Congress on Research in Burns.* Edinburgh, 20–24 September, 1965. Eds A. B. Wallace and A. W. Wilkinson, p. 12. Edinburgh: Livingstone

COPE, O. and MOORE, F. D. (1947) The redistribution of body water and the fluid therapy of the burned patient. *Annals of Surgery,* **126,** 1010

DAVIES, J. W. L. and TOPLEY, E. (1956) The disappearance of red cells in patients with burns. *Clinical Science (Oxford),* **15,** 135

DE WARDENER, H. E. (1969) Control of sodium reabsorption. *British Medical Journal,* **3,** 611, 676

DUDLEY, H. A. F., BATCHELOR, A. D. R. and SUTHERLAND, A. (1957) The management of haemoglobinuria in extensive burns. *British Journal of Plastic Surgery,* **9,** 275

EVANS, A. J. (1957) Experiences of a burns unit: A review of 520 cases. *British Medical Journal,* **2,** 547

EVANS, A. J. (1969) The treatment of burns shock. In *Pharmacological Treatment in Burns.* Eds A. Bertelli and L. Donati, p. 53. Amsterdam: Excerpta Medica

EVANS, E. I. and BIGGAR, I. A. (1945) The rationale of whole blood therapy in patients with burns. *Annals of Surgery,* **122,** 693

EVANS, E. I., PURNELL, O. J., BOBINETT, P. W., BATCHELOR, A. D. R. and MARTIN, M. (1952) Fluid and electrolyte requirements in severe burns. *Annals of Surgery,* **135,** 804

FLEAR, C. T. G., McNEILL, I. F., GREENER, J. S. and SINGH, C. M. (1969) Crystalloid administration in shock and surgical trauma. *Lancet,* **ii,** 155

GIBSON, T. and BROWN, A. (1945) Studies of burns and scalds. *Special Report Series of the Medical Research Council (London),* No. 249

GRÖNWALL, A. (1957) *Dextran and its Use in Colloidal Infusion Solutions.* Stockholm: Almqvist and Wiksell

HARDAWAY, R. M. (1968) The use of plasma expanders. *Hospital Medicine,* **2,** 1198

HARKINS, H. N. (1942) *The Treatment of Burns.* Springfield, Ill.: C. C. Thomas

HINTON, P. and ALLISON, S. P. (1969) Crystalloid administration in shock and surgical trauma. *Lancet,* **ii,** 594

JACKSON, D. McG. and CASON, J. S. (1966) The treatment of burns shock with oral hypotonic saline-bicarbonate solution. In *Research in Burns. Transactions of the Second International Congress in Research in Burns,* Edinburgh 1965, p. 61. Edinburgh: E. & S. Livingstone

KYLE, M. J. and WALLACE, A. B. (1951) Fluid replacement in burnt children. *British Journal of Plastic Surgery,* **3,** 194

LATIMER, R. D. (1971) Central venous catheterization. *British Journal of Hospital Medicine,* **5,** 369

LE QUESNE, L. P. (1957) *Fluid Balance in Surgical Practice,* 2nd edn. London: Lloyd-Luke (Medical Books)

MARKLEY, K., BOCANEGRA, M., BAZAN, A., TEMPLE, R., CHIAPPORI, M. and MORALES, G. (1956) Clinical evaluation of saline solution therapy in burn shock. I. *Journal of the American Medical Association,* **161,** 1465

MARKLEY, K., BOLANEGRA, M., BAZAN, A., TEMPLE, R., CHIAPPORI, M. and MORALES, G. (1959) Clinical evaluation of saline solution therapy in burn shock. II. *Journal of the American Medical Association,* **170,** 1633

MASTERTON, J. P. and DUDLEY, H. A. F. (1971) Balanced salt solution in burn shock – a re-appraisal. In *Research in Burns. Transactions of the Third International Congress in Research in Burns,* Prague 1970. Bern: Hans Huber

MONAFO, W. W. (1970) The treatment of burn shock by the intravenous and oral administration of hypertonic lactated solution. *Journal of Trauma,* **10,** 575

MORGAN, T. O. (1969) A study of some of the factors controlling sodium, potassium and water movement in the nephron using the technique of micro-perfusion. *MD thesis,* University of Sydney. Cited in de Wardener, H. E. (1973) In *Handbook of Physiology,* Section 8. Eds J. Orloff and R. W. Berliner. Washington DC: American Physiological Society

MOYER, C. A. (1953) An assessment of the therapy of burns. *Annals of Surgery,* **137,** 628

MOYER, C. A., MARGRAF, H. W. and MONAFO, W. N. Jr (1965) Burn shock and extravascular sodium deficiency – treatment with Ringer's solution with lactate. *Archives of Surgery,* **90,** 799

MOYER, C. A. and BUTCHER, H. R. (1967) *Burns, Shock, and Plasma Volume Regulations.* Saint Louis: C. V. Mosby

MUIR, I. F. K. (1961) Red cell destruction in burns. *British Journal of Plastic Surgery,* **14,** 273

MUIR, I. F. K. and JONES, P. F. (1976) Curling's ulcer: a rare condition. *British Journal of Surgery,* **63,** 60

NATIONAL RESEARCH COUNCIL (1943) *Burns, Shock, Wound Healing and Vascular Injuries* (Conference on Burns, 1942). Philadelphia: W. B. Saunders Co. Quoted by Cope and Moore (1947)

REISS, E., STIRMAN, J. A., ARTZ, C. P., DAVIS, J. H. and AMSPACHER, W. H. (1953) Fluid and electrolyte balance in burns. *Journal of the American Medical Association,* **152,** 1309

SETTLE, J. A. D. (1974) Urine output following severe burns. *Burns,* **1,** 23–42

SEVITT, S. (1956) Distal tubular necrosis with little or no oliguria. *Journal of Clinical Pathology,* **9,** 12

SEVITT, S. (1957) *Burns: Pathology and Therapeutic Applications,* p. 47. London: Butterworths

SØRENSEN, B. and SEJRSEN, P. (1965) Saline solutions in the treatment of burn shock. *Acta Chirurgica Scandinavica,* **129,** 239

SØRENSEN, B., SEJRSEN, P. and THOMSEN, M. (1967) Dextran solutions in the treatment of burn shock. *Scandinavian Journal of Plastic Reconstructive Surgery,* **1,** 68

SQUIRE, J. R., MAYCOCK, W. D'A., BULL, J. P. and RICKETTS, C. R. (1955) *Dextran: its Properties and Use in Medicine.* Oxford: Blackwell Scientific

STONE, H. H., RHAME, D. W., BLACK, W. S. and MARTIN, J. D. (1969) A universal burn solution: evaluation of initial intravenous fluid resuscitation. *Archives of Surgery,* **99,** 464

TOPLEY, E. and JACKSON, D. McG. (1957) The clinical control of red cell loss in burns. *Journal of Clinical Pathology,* **10,** 1

WILSON, W. C., MacGREGOR, A. R. and STEWART, C. P. (1938) The clinical course and pathology of burns and scalds under modern methods of treatment. *British Journal of Surgery,* **25,** 826

YU, H., COOPER, E. H., SETTLE, J. A. D. and MEADOWS, T. (1983) Urinary protein profiles after burn injury. *Burns,* **9,** 339–349

Chapter 3

Local treatment of the burn wound

There can be few conditions for which a greater number of different methods of treatment have been suggested than the wound produced by a burn.

The very number of different treatments available is a sure indication that no one method has any clear advantage over the others or is universally applicable, although the claims of some authors suggest that they would have us think otherwise.

The theoretical basis of the treatment of burn wounds is simple and all methods of treatment must conform with certain well-established principles of the natural history of burns.

It is therefore proposed firstly to state briefly these basic principles, and then to discuss in more detail the pathological processes and the choice and practical application of the different methods of treatment.

Summary of basic principles

Depth of burning

For all practical purposes the fate of an area of burned skin depends upon the depth of skin destruction at the time of the injury. The important distinction must be made between:

(*a*) Partial skin thickness burn.
(*b*) Whole skin thickness burn.

Natural history

Partial skin thickness burn
If infection can be prevented these will heal spontaneously. There is no known treatment which will improve this spontaneous healing, but bacterial infection can seriously interfere with healing and can convert a partial thickness burn into a full thickness burn.

The main aim of treatment is therefore to prevent infection.
An important distinction must be made between:

(*i*) Superficial partial thickness burn which will heal leaving no scarring.
(*ii*) Deep partial thickness burn which will heal but may do so with severe scarring.

Whole skin thickness burn

In the ordinary course of events the destroyed skin will separate as a slough leaving a raw area. It is the infection of this raw area which is the main cause of serious illness and death, and it is the fibrosis which develops in this raw area that is responsible for the contractures and deformities of burns.

In order to keep the danger period as short as possible and minimize the deformities, the aim of treatment is therefore:

(*i*) To get rid of destroyed skin as quickly as possible.
(*ii*) To get the raw area healed by skin grafting.

Four clinical types

With these points in mind four clinical types of burns can be recognized:

(*a*) The burn is obviously partial thickness – clearly conservative treatment only is indicated (*Plates 1* and *2a, see* opposite p. 1160)
(*b*) The burn is obviously whole thickness with clearly demarcated edges – often a contact burn. The treatment is removal of the slough as soon as possible (by surgical excision when feasible) and grafting (*Plates 2c* and *4a, see* opposite p. 60).
(*c*) In many serious burns it is impossible to say with certainty which areas are partial and which whole thickness destruction. The traditional pattern of treatment is therefore:

(*i*) Conservative treatment to prevent infection until the differentiation between partial and whole thickness burning can be made with certainty – usually 14 to 21 days.
(*ii*) Removal of slough as quickly as possible.
(*iii*) Closure of the raw surface by grafting (*Plates 3* and *4, see* opposite p. 60).

(*d*) Certain deep partial thickness burns pose special problems which require special methods of treatment (*Plate 2b, see* opposite p. 60).

These problems and the methods of achieving the objectives will now be discussed in detail.

Natural history – depth of burning

According to the circumstances of injury the severity of burning can vary from a simple erythema of the skin to deep charring with involvement of muscle and even bone, and the classification of Dupuytren into six stages, which is the best known of the older classifications, included burns of all severities.

In the majority of burns seen in clinical practice, however, the damage involves only skin and subcutaneous tissue, and from the point of view of treatment and prognosis the all-important distinction lies between burns in which:

(*a*) A partial thickness of the skin has been destroyed.
(*b*) The whole thickness of the skin has been destroyed.

These two groups represent the first and second degree burns of the classification which has been used for many years in Scotland (Department of Health, Scotland, 1942).

A classification involving three degrees is widely used, the three degrees corresponding to superficial partial thickness, deep partial thickness and whole thickness skin destruction.

The different classifications can be compared as follows:

(A)	(B) (Scotland)	(C) (USA)	(D)
Partial thickness skin destruction	1st degree	1st degree	Superficial partial thickness skin destruction
		2nd degree	Deep partial thickness skin destruction
Whole thickness skin destruction	2nd degree	3rd degree	Whole thickness skin destruction

The authors believe that the use of the numerical degrees, i.e. B and C above, has led to confusion in the past and should be abandoned. Either A or D, however, may be used as convenient and should be readily understood when transmitting information from one doctor to another.

The depth of these types of burns in relation to the layers of the skin is shown in *Figure 3.1*.

It must be remembered that this is a pathological classification and it is not possible to translate these depths of burning simply into clinical terms.

Superficial partial thickness burns

In all but the most superficial burns, the epidermis is completely destroyed but the hair follicles and sebaceous glands as well as the sweat glands are spared.

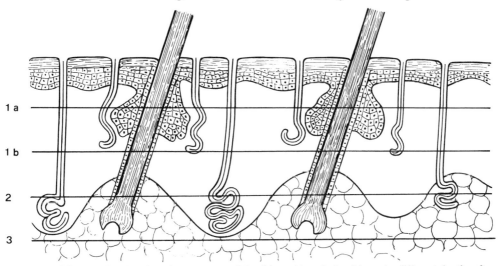

Figure 3.1 Diagram showing the microstructure of the skin and its relationship to the different depths of burning. Level 1A: superficial partial thickness burn passes through hair follicles, sebaceous glands and sweat glands. Level 1B: also superficial partial thickness burn, but deep to the sebaceous glands. It passes through hair roots and sweat glands. The dermis–fat interface is not breached. Level 2: deep partial thickness burn passes through hair roots and sweat glands, but breaches the dermis–fat interface and cuts across the fat domes. Level 3: full thickness burn passes deep to all epithelial structures.

At no place does the damage extend through the dermis–subcutaneous tissue interface. From the surviving epithelial structures, epithelium rapidly spreads to provide an intact epithelial surface, from which the superficial dead layers flake off revealing a skin which is elastic, supple and of excellent quality, and which in time may be indistinguishable from normal.

Deep partial thickness burns

A substantial part of the dermis and all sebaceous glands are destroyed and only the deeper parts of the hair follicles or the sweat glands survive, the relative numbers and depth of these structures varying in different parts of the body. A critical factor is that, because the dermis–subcutaneous interface is not flat, the margin of tissue destruction extends into the subcutaneous tissue at the places where this pushes up into the dermis (the so-called 'fat domes'). This depth of burning can often be recognized at the stage of separation of slough and is sometimes referred to by the alternative name of 'deep dermal burn'.

Even the small surviving scraps of epithelium suffice for re-epithelialization of the surface, but this is much slower than in the previous type and the healed skin is imperfect and often shows hypertrophic scarring.

Whole thickness burns

When the full thickness of the skin has been destroyed and there are no surviving epithelial elements, the sequence of events is quite different and the position is much more serious.

In the absence of infection, the area of destroyed skin becomes dry, hard and black – the characteristic slough of a full thickness burn.

In the surviving tissue immediately underneath the slough, cellular and capillary activity produces a layer of granulation tissue, and the enzymatic activity of this layer loosens the slough which finally comes away, exposing the red surface of the granulations.

Since the granulations contain no epithelial cells, healing of the area can only occur by ingrowth of cells from the surviving epithelial edge. Initially this is rapid, but as the epithelium grows further and further away from its original site, it grows more and more slowly until finally it stops altogether and occasionally an ungrafted burn may be seen still unhealed even after 15 or 20 years.

While these events are taking place on the surface, changes are also taking place in the granulation tissue. In the deeper layers collagen is laid down. There is reduction in vascularity, and finally the tissue becomes a scar tissue. At the same time, the superficial layers of granulation tissue ooze serum which clots and is itself invaded by cells and capillaries to form fresh granulation tissue.

As long as the surface remains unepithelialized there is thus a continuous process of laying down of fresh granulation tissue on the surface, while the deeper layers progressively mature into scar tissue.

As soon as the scar tissue is formed, it begins to contract with tremendous force, shrinking to only a fraction of its original size. It is this contraction of scar tissue which is the cause of the deformities of severe burns, and it is the aim of the surgeon to epithelialize these raw areas by skin grafting, and thus to limit and cut short the formation of scar (*Figure 3.2*).

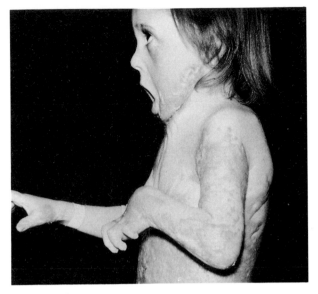

Figure 3.2 Crippling contracture in full thickness burns of neck and arm which has not been skin grafted

So long as the area remains raw it is liable to invasion by bacteria with their harmful local and general effects, and finally the raw area is a constant source of loss of protein and red cells, which places a severe drain on the patient's resources.

Bacterial infection

In spite of recent improvements in antibacterial substances, bacterial infection of the wound is still the single most important problem of the treatment of these patients.

The large raw area with its exudate of serum is like a huge culture plate on which organisms can multiply, little affected by the body defence mechanisms.

Some degree of bacterial contamination of the surface is almost inevitable, but is not necessarily incompatible with satisfactory healing of the burn if the body defences can match the virulence of the organisms.

In other instances, however, either because of great virulence of the organisms, or lowered body resistance, the balance may be upset, and local and general damage may occur.

Infection can cause trouble in the following ways:

(1) Local healing may be delayed.
(2) Viable epithelial cells may be killed, and a partial thickness defect may be converted into a full thickness defect.
(3) The 'take' of grafts may be jeopardized.
(4) Bacterial toxins may be absorbed causing general symptoms.
(5) Bacteria may invade deeper tissues causing cellulitis.
(6) Bacteria may gain entry to the blood stream causing septicaemia.

The following organisms have to be considered:

Streptococcus β-haemolyticus
Staphylococcus pyogenes (aureus)
Pseudomonas aeruginosa (pyocyanea)
Proteus vulgaris
Clostridium tetani
Eschericia coli
Klebsiella sp.

In days gone by β-haemolytic streptococcus was the most serious threat and investigations in the burns ward of the Glasgow Royal Infirmary showed that almost all burned patients admitted to hospital became infected with this organism at some stage of their stay in hospital (Cruickshank, 1935; Colebrook *et al.*, 1945). The haemolytic streptococcus is unrivalled in its power to kill surviving skin cells and to destroy skin grafts.

The advent of, first, sulphonamides, and then penicillin curbed the power of the streptococcus and, since the organism has shown no propensity to develop resistance to penicillin, it is easily controlled and has ceased to be a serious menace.

The organisms which are now responsible for most trouble in burns are *Staphylococcus pyogenes* and the Gram-negative organisms *Pseudomonas aeruginosa* and *Proteus vulgaris*.

Staphylococcus pyogenes is so widespread in hospitals that it is exceptional for a burn of any severity to run its course without being colonized with this organism sooner or later. Fortunately, it does not always cause serious trouble. In many instances, particularly in minor burns, the body defences seem to be able to come to terms with the organism, healing takes place without setbacks and grafts take successfully.

In other instances, the body defences fail to match the virulence of the organisms which invade healthy tissues with resultant harm to the patient. During the invasive phase, the bacteria can be attacked by antibiotics and in the early days of penicillin when staphylococci were sensitive to the drug, it seemed that one of the major problems had been solved.

Unfortunately, the organisms soon became resistant to penicillin and to each new antibiotic as it was introduced, and staphylococcal infection remained a serious problem. However, the advent of the semisynthetic penicillins (e.g. cloxacillin, ampicillin), fusidic acid, cephaloridine and the kanamycin group has provided a further range of drugs, and it is now seldom that the invasive effects of staphylococcal infection cannot be controlled. If the systemic effects are controlled, the local effects are usually not serious and it is only occasionally that a staphylococcus is encountered which will seriously interfere with the take of skin grafts.

Gram-negative bacteria, of which *Pseudomonas aeruginosa* is the most important, have been the most troublesome organisms of recent years (Barclay, 1970), but the re-introduction of silver nitrate and the advent of sulfamylon, gentamicin and silver sulphadiazine have improved the situation dramatically.

The Gram-negative organisms cause trouble in three different ways. (*a*) They produce a large quantity of pus containing toxins. The toxins may kill surviving skin cells and thus convert an initially partial thickness burn into a full thickness burn, and absorption of toxins may cause general illness. (*b*) The large quantity of pus produced may float off grafts and cause great difficulty in getting them to take.

(c) The invasive properties of these organisms are generally considered to be low, but a large burn causes such debility that septicaemia can easily occur, especially with *Pseudomonas aeruginosa*, and this condition will be fatal unless it is treated energetically.

Infections by other organisms are, in general, not very harmful and are of no special significance, but it is of interest to note that now that serious staphylococcal and pseudomonas infections are much less frequent following the introduction of the drugs mentioned above, the presence of *E. coli* and *Klebsiella sp., Bacteroides sp., Candida albicans* and other yeasts and fungi, become much more frequent in the bacteriological reports of cultures from burns wounds.

Tetanus occasionally appears in burns but in our experience this infection has occurred only in patients injured on farms.

Sources and modes of infection

Starting with the classical work of Lister (1867), a great deal of information has been accumulated about the modes of conveyance of pathogenic bacteria, and in recent years the work of Colebrook and Lowbury and their colleagues is noteworthy (Colebrook *et al.*, 1945; Colebrook, 1950; Cason and Lowbury, 1960; Lowbury, 1960).

Burns are sterile immediately after infliction, but are liable to be colonized very rapidly by bacteria. They may be infected from the hands or respiratory tracts of first-aiders, and there is a very high risk if patients are wrapped in unsterilized blankets.

In hospital practice the majority of organisms originate from other patients in the vicinity. If a patient acquires an organism in his wound, within a short space of time it can be found in his dressings, his clothes and his bed-clothes. From these sites the organisms may be transferred directly through the air to other patients or transmitted indirectly by the hands, arms and clothes of nurses and doctors (Barclay, 1970, 1971). Hospital staff may carry streptococci in their throats, particularly after suffering from 'colds', and they may also harbour staphylococci in their noses.

Less commonly the patient's burn may be infected by organisms which originate in his own nose and throat.

Clinical diagnosis of depth of burning

When patients are first seen an attempt should be made to assess the depth of the burn in terms of partial or full thickness destruction. This is sometimes easy, but often very difficult.

The temperature of the burning agent and the time of the exposure determine both the depth of burning and the appearance of the skin surfaces seen soon after the injury. As Jackson (1953) has pointed out, the appearance of the skin surface is a measure of the intensity of the heat stimulus, and does not always give reliable information about the depth of burning, e.g. a very high temperature for a short time may produce scorching of the surface of the skin, yet deeper layers may be intact. Nevertheless the appearance of the burn will usually allow at least a tentative assessment to be made. At this stage some burns will be obviously superficial, some obviously deep, and some of doubtful depth, and in some burns areas of the three types will be present.

Simple erythema is always indicative of superficial damage, and blistering is usually so. In other cases the superficial layers of the skin are lost and the deeper layers are pink and viable, indicating partial thickness loss only (*Plate 2a, see* opposite p. 60).

At the other end of the scale the burn which is dark brown or black and leathery hard, and has a translucent appearance with thrombosed vessels seen through it, certainly involves the full thickness of the skin (*Plate 2c, see* opposite p. 60). Other appearances suggesting full thickness destruction are the brownish-yellow scorched skin with a dead white background, and also the dead white skin without scorching which is usually due to prolonged exposure to a relatively low temperature (*Plate 2b, see* opposite p. 60). This dead white skin can sometimes be mistakenly thought to be normal, but close inspection will reveal its abnormal pallor and loss of elasticity. This appearance is usually associated with a burn of deep partial thickness depth which can be expected to heal with a poor scar, but sometimes healing is good and scarring is minimal and sometimes the burn turns out to be of full thickness depth and grafting is necessary.

The appearance which causes most difficulty is the mottled red and white appearance with loss of the superficial layers of the skin (*Plate 2b, see* opposite p. 60). The redness is not affected by pressure, and is due to diapedesis of red cells through the damaged dermal capillaries. In general, the thicker the skin showing this appearance the more likely is it that some viable epithelial elements remain. Such a burn on the back may heal, whereas a burn of similar appearance on the front of the chest may not.

Pinprick test

Since the sensory end organs are concentrated in the skin, it follows that the presence of sensation indicates that part of the skin is still viable, while absence of sensation suggests whole thickness skin destruction. Touch is unsuitable as a form of sensation for testing, but the presence of pain on pricking with a pin is valuable evidence of the existence of a viable layer of the skin (Jackson, 1953).

The test is performed by pricking the skin firmly with a sterile pin or needle. The test is positive if the patient complains of feeling pain. For the test to be negative, it must be possible to drive the pin right through the skin into the subcutaneous fat without causing pain.

A positive reaction to pinprick is definite evidence of the presence of viable cells, but a negative reaction cannot be interpreted so firmly because, particularly in areas with a naturally low sensitivity, the pin can be driven right through the skin into the subcutaneous fat without causing pain, yet viable skin cells are still present and the skin will heal. The skin of the face is particularly liable to behave in this way.

Many other special methods have been used in order to try to assess the depth of burning, for example, temperature measurements, thermography, intravital dye injections, and isotope uptake, but none of these methods has been found to be consistently reliable or widely applicable. A reliable and practical method of determining the depth of a skin burn is still badly needed.

Conservative treatment directed towards the prevention of infection

All methods and variations of conservative treatment fall under the headings of either: (*a*) exposure treatment, or (*b*) treatment by dressings.

In many instances it will be found that treatment is not ideal by either of these methods, but that the one chosen is the best compromise available when all the prevailing factors have been considered. Furthermore, the use of one method does not compromise the surgeon as far as the other is concerned, and a method which is suitable at one stage of the evolution of a burn may be superseded by another at a later stage (*see Plate 4e-g,* opposite p. 60).

Exposure treatment

This is the most 'natural' method of treatment. It is of great antiquity but its popularity in its present form is due to the efforts of Wallace of Edinburgh (1949, 1951, 1952). The burned part, after being cleaned, is exposed to the air with no covering. The exudate dries and, with the layers of destroyed skin, forms a scab.*
This scab now protects the underlying tissues from contamination and beneath it healing can progress.

The method depends upon the conditions of: (*a*) dryness, (*b*) coolness, and (*c*) exposure to light, at the burn surface – conditions which are inimical to bacterial growth.

There is, of course, no mechanical barrier to infection, and under ordinary ward conditions some degree of bacterial contamination of the burn during the initial drying-out period is inevitable. Pathogenic organisms can be grown from the deep surfaces of apparently satisfactory crusts, but under the conditions of successful exposure the activity of these organisms is so limited that the body defences can deal with them, and healing can take place.

There is evidence that the drying process may result in marginal increase in the depth of tissue destruction and there is no doubt that separation of the slough by a natural enzymatic process and subsequent spread of epithelium is more rapid under moist than under dry conditions, but the damage caused by bacterial infection is so much more harmful than the effects of dryness that under certain conditions exposure treatment remains a good compromise.

Exposure treatment is particularly suitable for:

(*a*) Single surface burns of trunk or limbs.
(*b*) Burns of face.
(*c*) Burns near the perineum.
(*d*) Extensive and complicated burns which cannot be adequately dressed.

Preliminary treatment
In minor burns which do not require transfusion, treatment can be instituted as soon as the patient is seen. In burns serious enough to require transfusion, shock must be brought under control before local treatment is started. General anaesthesia is not necessary, and the treatment can be carried out under sedation by morphine, which may be the initial dose as described in the section on shock treatment or, if treatment has to be delayed more than four hours, a second dose may be given.

The burn is cleaned gently by a warm cetrimide–chlorhexidine solution (e.g. Savlon), all loose skin is removed, blisters snipped, the fluid removed and the overlying skin excised. The area is then left exposed to the air. No antibiotic or other powder is applied to the burn. Various substances have been recommended

---

* The term 'eschar' is sometimes used for the scab.

for application to the surface to inhibit bacteria, but most of these have proved to have some disadvantages. Organic iodine preparations are the best available at the moment and may be applied either in an aerosol spray or as an ointment.

If exposure treatment is to work satisfactorily it must be possible to expose the burn surface completely. This is easy to arrange for burns of only one surface of trunk or limbs, but with ingenuity its use can be extended to more extensive and complicated areas.

It is also of value, if the burn involves the neighbourhood of a joint, to apply some form of splintage to prevent cracks developing in the crust.

Progress

Once a satisfactory crust has formed it is inspected every day, particular care being taken to observe any cracks developing. After about a week the crust begins to separate at the edge and this loose edge is lifted gently and snipped away with scissors.

In the neighbourhood of joints, cracks easily develop in the crust if the area cannot be immobilized, and infection may enter via the cracks. Ideally, the eschar should remain supple and attempts are being made to find some method of plasticizing it. Some success has been obtained by painting the eschar with glycerin.

If the burn is entirely partial thickness the whole scab will finally be removed leaving an intact skin surface (*Plate 1c* and *d, see* opposite p. 60). If, however, there is a central area of full thickness burning, separation will cease and this central area will remain static for some days.

If the scab has not separated by 21 days it should be assumed that it covers an area of full thickness burning, and the treatment should therefore be changed to a method designed to encourage separation of the slough (*see below*).

Circumferential burns

These burns pose a problem because of the difficulty of exposing opposite sides of the limb or trunk. Opposite sides can be exposed alternatively by using a special turning frame (e.g. Circ-o-lectric) which enables the patient to be turned frequently without being actually handled. Ventilating frames were described by Evans of Roehampton (1957), and consist of a net of nylon stretched tightly on a rectangular metal structure. The netting is too hard for the patient to lie on in comfort and a layer of polyurethane foam covers the nylon net. This provided a soft and non-adherent bed for the patient and because of the porosity of the material some ventilation takes place through its substance. Even better ventilation could take place if the foam layer could be omitted, but so far no material has been found which is strong enough to support the patient's weight, yet still sufficiently soft and pliable for him to lie on in comfort.

Other special beds incorporating an air flow system are described below.

Air conditioning – control of microclimate

Exposure treatment may fail either if there is an unusually large number of bacteria in the air to which the patient is exposed or if drying of the exposed surface is so much delayed that even a few bacteria can colonize the surface and multiply (Barclay and Dexter, 1968). An additional problem of exposure treatment is that evaporation of exudate results in loss of heat from the patient and he may go through a phase of heat imbalance.

For these reasons, modern air engineering techniques have been invoked in order to manipulate the patient's environment – often referred to as the 'microclimate' – to best advantage (Muir and Stranc, 1966).

The present evidence makes it certain that air-borne infection of burns arises from particles carried by air currents from the floor or other surfaces and from particles shed by the skin of nurses and doctors and other attendants.

It should, therefore, in theory be possible and indeed it has been shown to be possible in practice to prevent contamination of the burn by:

(1) Enclosing the patient in a ventilated plastic tent with special arrangements for nursing procedures.
(2) Or a combination of:

   (a) Surrounding the patient with a high speed stream of filtered air (often referred to as a laminar flow system although air does not flow in a truly laminar fashion).
   (b) Dressing all attendants in bacteria proof clothing and preferably with a body exhaust system.

In practice these systems have been found to be impracticable and it has been necessary to accept compromise solutions the main features of which are:

(1) Good conventional air conditioning with filtered bacteria-proof air of the same standard as is used in operating theatres, i.e. approximately 20 changes per hour.
(2) The use of special beds with an in-built air system.
(3) The use of light comfortable bacteria-proof clothing for the attendants.

Special beds
These all have a supply of filtered air and have the great advantage that it is easy to control the patient's microclimate in terms of temperature and humidity.

The only bed which gives complete exposure to circumferential burns is the levitation 'high loss' air bed which works on a hovercraft principle, but there have been practical difficulties with this and it has not yet been accepted for general use (Scales *et al.*, 1967; Sanders, Scales and Muir, 1970).

The 'low loss' air bed is excellent for comfort and ease of handling but the patient lies on impermeable material and must therefore be turned.

The 'clinitron' bed (*Figure 3.3*) consists of a sand-like mass of tiny beads which is made into a quicksand consistency by air flow, thereby avoiding excess pressure to any one point.

The Howorth climator (*Figure 3.4*) consists of a ventilated polyurethane mattress with a self-contained air supply unit. This has great advantages of simplicity and mobility but ventilation of the body surface taking weight is only partial and patients with circumferential burns need to be turned.

Clothing for doctors and nurses
Good disposable or semidisposable suits are now available made of material which is permeable to air and therefore comfortable to wear but prevents passage of bacteria-carrying particles (*see Figure 3.5*).

It is essential that the trousers should be closed at the ankles to prevent particles from the perineum of the wearer being swept out by air currents.

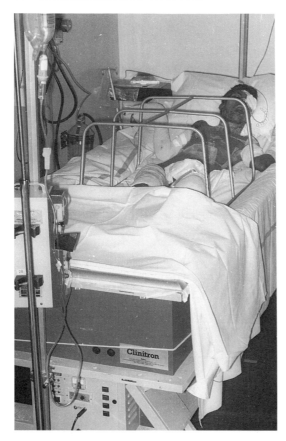

Figure 3.3 'Clinitron' fluidized bead bed in use. Pressure areas are protected by wide distribution of the load

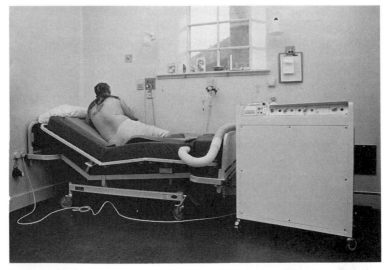

Figure 3.4 Howorth climator for exposure treatment. The console provides a floor of air with temperature and humidity control. The thin upper part of the mattress, of permeable polyurethane foam, is changed daily and can be autoclaved

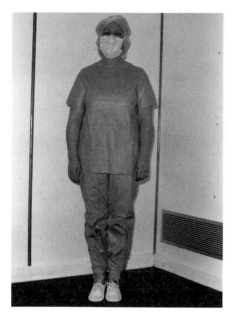

Figure 3.5 Surgikos disposable clothing for nurses and medical staff in burns rooms. The material is non-woven and does not allow passage of bacteria-carrying particles. Note closure of trousers at ankles

Heat loss and temperature control

The evaporation of surface water which is an essential feature of the exposure treatment results in substantial heat losses which, in spite of a great deal of investigation, has not yet been accurately measured.

The ability to control the patient's microclimate makes it possible to compensate for these losses. This has been done mainly by warming the ambient air, but recent work suggests that it may not be possible to achieve adequate compensation by air convection and it may be necessary to use radiant heat.

If radiant heat is not used the air temperature needs to be in the range of 80–90 °F but this will depend on the rate of air flow and the humidity. With orthodox rates of air flow, i.e. in a conventional air-conditioned room, 40 per cent humidity will give satisfactory drying; although most patients will be comfortable in this climate some will still complain of feeling cold.

Treatment by dressings – theoretical background

The purposes of dressings are:

(1) To provide a mechanical barrier to prevent bacteria-carrying particles from alighting on the wound.
(2) To absorb fluid exudate.
(3) To act as a vehicle for antibacterial substances.

Over the years there has been a shift of emphasis from one of these functions to another, and a further change has occurred again recently.

Prior to the introduction of antiseptics by Lister in 1967 the absorption of fluid exudate was considered the most important function of the dressing. The leading exponents of this view were Syme (1837) and Samson Gamgee (1876) who maintained that the dryness at the wound surface produced by an absorptive dressing diminished the chances of the wound becoming septic. Although they were, at that time, ignorant of the bacterial nature of infection, subsequent work has confirmed the correctness of their observations; they must, however, have had failures, since their dressings were not aseptic. When Lister first introduced his antiseptic treatment with carbolic acid, he was much concerned with the maintenance of a high concentration of the antiseptic at the surface of the wound, and in order to achieve this he made repeated applications of the carbolic acid to the inner dressing. Absorption of wound secretions was considered to be of secondary importance. Unfortunately carbolic acid, and indeed all the early antiseptics, were unselective in their action, and killed normal tissue cells as well as the bacteria. While this might be acceptable at the relatively small surface of a wound due to mechanical trauma, the tissue damage caused over the wide area of a burn was a serious drawback, and the results of antiseptic treatment of burns were disappointing. For this reason there was a swing back to the principles advocated by Gamgee, using a bland inner dressing such a paraffin-impregnated tulle gras covered by a massive absorptive dressing of gauze and cotton wool. Now, however, the dressings were presterilized, thus minimizing the chances of superadded infection. When sulphonamides and later penicillin and other antibiotics became available, these were added to the inner layer of the dressing which was then covered by an absorptive layer, thus apparently combining the advantages of the two methods – absorption and antisepsis. It was thought that the undisturbed dressing formed a good mechanical barrier against infection and that the risk of contamination was great only at the time of change of dressing. Furthermore, it was expected that the antibacterial substance in the inner layer would retain its potency for many days. For these reasons, the dressings were changed infrequently, for example only every 7 days or so. It now seems likely that these views were unduly optimistic. Infection often appeared in burns treated by dressings applied skilfully and under good conditions, and even when the outer layers of the dressings remained dry. During the first two or three days when the burn is in a state of rapid exudation, the antiseptic is so diluted or washed away that it is effective for only 24 or even 12 hours after it has been applied. On the other hand, there is now some evidence that if the antiseptic is changed frequently, even if this does increase the chances of contamination at dressing times, the rate of infection is reduced (Muir, Owen and Murphy, 1969). So the requirement, in burns treatment as so often elsewhere, is to choose from a number of different techniques, and to try to select the method which best fits the particular circumstances. In some of these circumstances the absorptive dressing with an inner antiseptic layer changed relatively infrequently will be appropriate. In other cases, however, and particularly with extensive burns being treated by some of the newer potent antiseptics, a technique which involves frequent changes of the antiseptic, with minimal dressings, is more suitable.

Materials for dressings
The properties of a satisfactory absorptive dressing must be such that it can absorb an adequate amount of fluid and distribute the fluid evenly throughout its substance so that pooling does not occur. The material which best fulfils these criteria is cotton gauze. Pads made entirely of gauze are the most satisfactory absorbent dressings at present available. These are not prepared commercially and must therefore be 'homemade'. The necessary thickness may be made up by a

number of flat layers, but a more satisfactory method is to use a mass of fluffed gauze in a sandwich between two flat layers of gauze as in the Brooke Army dressing (Davis *et al.*, 1953).

Dressings of this type can be prepared beforehand in suitable sizes for individual patients.

Because of the high cost of gauze the most commonly used absorptive dressing comprises an inner layer of gauze and an outer layer of cotton wool. Cotton wool is cheaper than gauze but it is not such an efficient absorptive and fluid tends to pool in the dressing rather than be distributed evenly throughout its fabric.

Gamgee tissue, which is a sandwich of cotton wool between two sheets of gauze, is useful because of its ease of handling and because it is produced in suitably large sizes. Its absorptive capacity is that of the wool which composes most of its bulk.

Inner layer
In the early stages the inner layer of dressing will contain an antiseptic. In addition, because of the tendency of dressings to stick to burn wounds, with subsequent pain and tissue trauma when the dressing is removed, it is an obvious advantage if the inner layer is non-adherent. Many commercial preparations are available, most of which consist of tulle gras – a wide mesh gauze – impregnated with an antiseptic in a base either of paraffin or a water-miscible cream. These gauzes are acceptably non-adherent as long as they are not allowed to dry out. Alternatively, the antiseptic made up in a suitable cream can be spread by hand on sheets of cotton gauze which are then applied to the wound. Various other materials such as perforated plastic sheeting or sponge-like foamed plastic have been tried but have not proved generally satisfactory.

Outer layer – pressure bandages
When the absorptive dressing has been applied it is fixed in place with a bandage. Crepe bandages, because of the way they conform to the contour of the body, are undoubtedly most satisfactory, but are very expensive. Cotton and conforming bandages (Kling bandage) have some use but are not satisfactory if placed over joints. On the trunk many-tailed bandages are often useful.

Some mention should be made here of the place of 'pressure bandaging' and 'pressure dressings'. The notion that the application of firm pressure on a wound is beneficial is of long standing and was stressed, among others, by Sampson Gamgee (1876) who stated: 'There must be no constriction – only equable adaption of surface to surface with the light pressure which always comforts. There must be no squeezing like that of an old college friend's hand when seen after long absence; such pressure as that, if continued, is intolerable constriction. The soothing surgical pressure is like that which you interchange with the hand of a lady, the pleasure of whose meeting is tempered by the respectable regard which she inspires.'

The bandage should certainly hold the dressing in firm contact with the burn, so as to facilitate absorption of the discharge, and there is no reason to doubt that, in the limbs, sufficient pressure can be exerted to limit the amount of swelling which occurs after a burn and, particularly in the hand, this may be of value in expediting recovery of function. There is, however, no convincing evidence that pressure bandaging can influence the fate of an area of burned skin, nor that it can reduce the amount of oedema sufficiently to influence the development of shock. It should be remembered that over a large part of the body surface (face, neck and trunk), it is virtually impossible to apply even pressure for any length of time by means of bandages.

We conclude, therefore, that bandages should indeed be applied so as to exert even pressure whenever possible, but that the merits of 'pressure dressings' have been exaggerated.

It is important that the outer layers should be porous to allow evaporation of water, indeed the whole dressing has been described as an 'evaporating dressing'. Attempts to prevent fluid coming through the dressing by incorporating an impervious layer result in the dressing becoming soggy and encourage bacterial growth.

It will also be apparent that, in circumferential burns, the side of the body or limb which is underneath will tend to become soggy and arrangements must be made to ventilate this as with a burn being treated by exposure.

The dressing itself acts as padding and the dressed part can therefore lie on the netting of the frame. Any parts not padded by dressing can be protected by sections of polyurethane foam.

Turning frames can also be used to give ventilation of alternate sides.

Antibacterial substances for inclusion in the dressing
It will be remembered that the early wound dressings used by Lister were antiseptic dressings, and the idea of using inert sterile dressings was a later development.

Immediately after being burned, the surface of the skin is sterile and the only organisms present are those deep in skin glands, which are of low pathogenicity. Some organisms will usually alight on the burn between its occurrence and the application of the first dressing, but it should theoretically be possible to kill these by a suitable antiseptic, and then prevent further infection by a simple sterile dressing. Practical experience, however, shows that under these conditions infection frequently occurs. The presence of discharged serum in the dressing and on the skin surface, the warmth, and lack of light under the dressing all provide an ideal environment for organisms. It needs only a few organisms to gain entrance along the skin surface or through the dressing to result in a substantial infection. If the dressing becomes soaked through to the outside the entrance of organisms is greatly facilitated, and can take place in a very short space of time.

The earlier antiseptics used, such as carbolic acid, mercurial compounds and aniline dyes, had the disadvantage that their action was unselective, causing damage to surviving tissue cells, as well as to bacteria, and therefore often did as much harm as good.

Sulphonamide was the first substance to have a strong action against bacteria without a toxic effect on tissue cells, and was shown by Colebrook and his colleagues (1945) to be very successful in reducing infection by haemolytic streptococci. When penicillin became available, this was also shown to have a powerful action against streptococci and in addition against staphylococci. Unfortunately, it was not long before many strains of staphylococci appeared which were resistant to the action of penicillin and, as new antibiotics were developed and used, this same problem of resistant strains of staphylococci recurred. The commonly used antibiotics – the penicillins, the tetracyclines and others – had the added disadvantage that they possessed little or no inhibiting action on Gram-negative organisms. A number of antibiotics and antiseptics were produced which were not suitable for systemic use but were suitable for local application. Most of these – gramicidin, neomycin, bacitracin, polymyxin, framycetin, nitrofurazone, chlorhexidine – had the advantage that organisms did not develop resistance to them. These substances have all been used singly and in various combinations. They have proved useful in the past and many of them are still useful under certain circumstances. However, they all failed to prevent serious infection in extensive burns, and none gave satisfactory protection against *Pseudomonas* which for a long period has been the main source of anxiety in burns units. The search therefore continued for more suitable antiseptics which would be active against Gram-negative organisms as well as against Gram-positive organisms. In 1965, Moyer and colleagues showed that excellent prophylaxis against *Pseudomonas* and other organisms could be achieved by using dressings which were kept continuously wet with a 0.5 per cent solution of silver nitrate. This treatment, however, had certain disadvantages. It was prophylactic only and did not control established infection; there was a loss of electrolytes which required to be made good by electrolyte supplements; some patients complained of discomfort from lying in a continuously wet environment; the silver nitrate caused black staining of the patient, the bedclothes and the nurses.

Sulfamylon (Mafenide), introduced in 1964 (Lindberg *et al.*, 1965), superseded silver nitrate in most centres. Sulfamylon is a sulphonamide derivative which has been known since the early 1940s, but was not then extensively investigated because it was found to be relatively inactive against Gram-positive organisms, particularly streptococci, which at that time were the main cause of trouble. It does, however, have a strong action against *Pseudomonas*, and not only is it effective in prophylaxis, but it also diffuses readily into tissues without loss of potency and is thus effective in the treatment of established infections. Disadvantages are that it sometimes causes severe pain and that it is relatively ineffective against Gram-positive organisms, although experience suggests that this is more obvious *in vitro* than *in vivo*, and in fact staphylococcal infection has not been a serious problem in patients treated with sulfamylon.

Silver sulphadiazine cream was introduced as an antiseptic for application to burns by Fox in 1968, and after nearly two decades of very widespread use no serious side-effects have been reported.

Topical application of gentamicin, a powerful antibiotic effective against both Gram-positive and Gram-negative organisms, has found favour in many centres, but in the authors' view this drug should be reserved exclusively for systemic use, in circumstances described on page 108.

Mode of incorporation of antiseptics in the dressing
The purpose of antiseptics in the dressing is two-fold: first, to control any organisms on the surface of the burn and, secondly, to deal with organisms in the substance of the dressing so as to prevent ingress of new organisms from the exterior and also to reduce dissemination of the patient's own organisms into the environment. The problem was clearly defined by Lord Lister and his final solution involved the use of two antiseptics (Lister, 1907). He used 1:40 carbolic acid on the inner layer of dressing in contact with the wound. This was rapidly bactericidal on the surface of the wound, but because of its solubility, was only short-acting. The outer layers of dressing were impregnaged with the double cyanide of zinc and mercury. The relatively insoluble compound was fixed in the fibres of the dressing by a dye, rosaniline, which gave the gauze its characteristic blue colour. The dressing therefore contained a reservoir of cyanide which continually dissolved in the discharge and maintained a bacteriostatic concentration. About the efficacy of an inner antiseptic layer there is general agreement, but much less attention has been paid to the use of antiseptics in the main bulk of the dressings. Lowbury and Hood

(1952) showed how rapidly organisms could pass through dressings and plaster casts, and they reported trials of dressings impregnated with an organic mercury compound. Good results were reported but they do not seem to have pursued the matter further. The mercurial antiseptics suggested by Lister have been avoided because of possible toxic effects, although the actual evidence of this is small; there is a need for further trials of dressings impregnated with newer antiseptics.

The antiseptics available
Many different antiseptic preparations are available. The following list is not exhaustive but contains those preparations which have been used consistently in our departments.

Chlorhexidine (Hibitane)   This is a good general purpose antiseptic which is active against Gram-positive but not Gram-negative organisms. It is available in an impregnated paraffin gauze (Bactigras) and is suitable for use particularly in smaller burns and burns which are not expected to exude much.

Silver sulphadiazine (Flamazine, Silvadine)   This is available as a cream and is probably the most widely used antiseptic for severe burns at the present moment. It has a wide antibacterial range effective against both Gram-positive and Gram-negative organisms. Bacterial resistance does not develop and there are few sensitivity reactions.
   Although it is effective in prophylaxis of pseudomonas infections it is not as good as sulfamylon for treatment of established infections.
   Its main disadvantage is that it alters the appearance of the surface of the burn which often looks unhealthy even when progress is good, and it becomes impossible to tell the depth of the burn. It is not therefore suitable if any form of early surgery is contemplated.

Sulfamylon (Mafenide)   This is not active against Gram-positive organisms and has therefore been superceded by silver sulphadiazine for general use. It remains the best antiseptic for treatment of established pseudomonas infection. It is available as a cream. In a substantial proportion of cases it causes severe pain and its use has then to be discontinued.

Silver nitrate   This is used as a 0.5 per cent aqueous solution with which gauze dressings are kept continually wet. Although it has a marked prophylactic effect against infection, it is not as good as other preparations for treatment of established infection. At the moment its practical disadvantages, in particular the dark staining of the environment and the prolonged discomfort of continuous wet application, seem to outweigh the advantages.

Organic iodine preparations (povidone-iodine – Betadine)   These are available either as an aerosol spray or in an ointment base.

NPC cream   This is a cream containing neomycin, chlorhexidine and polymyxins (Cason and Lowbury, 1960).

Neomycin sulphate	2 mg
Chlorhexidine dihydrochloride	1 mg

Polymyxin B   1 mg
Cetomacrogol 1000 emulsifying wax (BPC) to   1 g

The neomycin and chlorhexidine are active against streptococci and staphylococci and the polymyxin against *Pseudomonas pyocyanea*. It is not available
commercially and, since the ingredients are not heat stable, it cannot be
incorporated in gauze and autoclaved, but must be prepared under sterile
conditions and spread on to gauze by hand or with a spatula before use. It is not as
effective against *Pseudomonas* as sulfamylon, but it is still a good broad-spectrum
preparation suitable for use in serious burns.

Dressing techniques
Antiseptic dressings may be used in one of two ways, according to the
circumstances.

Absorptive dresing with an inner antiseptic layer   This is suitable for burns of up to
10 per cent, which can be completely covered by the dressing, which should extent
for 10 cm (4 inches) beyond the margins of the burn at all points. This dressing
needs to be changed relatively infrequently. Any suitable convenient antiseptic
preparation can be used for the inner dressing.

Single layer antiseptic dressings without absorptive layer   This is suitable for
extensive burns over 10 per cent and can also be used for burns of any size
extending near the mouth, nose or perineum. The dressing must be changed
frequently. Sulfamylon, and silver sulphadiazine are the best antiseptics to use with
this technique.

Technique for treatment by antiseptic absorptive dressing

First dressing   The first dressing should be applied as soon as the patient's general
condition is satisfactory. All manipulations must be performed gently and a general
anaesthetic is not required, but sedation by morphine is helpful.

(*a*) The burn is cleaned with a cetrimide–chlorhexidine solution (e.g. Savlon). All
    loose skin is removed and blisters are snipped, the fluid evacuated and
    overlying skin removed.
(*b*) The area is then covered by a single layer of antiseptic tulle, four layers of
    gauze and a layer of cotton wool, and this is secured by a crepe bandage.
        Care is taken that the wool extends for a handsbreadth (=4 inches or 10 cm)
    beyond the edge of the burn.

First three days   The dressing should be inspected every day taking particular care
to observe if exudate has soaked through to the outer surface. If this has occurred,
the bandage and wool should be removed and fresh wool and bandage applied. The
amount of exudate which the dressing has to absorb is greatest during the first three
days and by the end of this time the dressing will be saturated with a protein-rich
fluid which, in spite of any antiseptics present, will be highly susceptible to
colonization by stray bacteria. The dressing should therefore be entirely changed at
the end of three days, the technique of application being similar to that of the first
dressing except that there is no need for any cleaning. The old dressing should be
removed and the new one should be applied immediately. If the burn is such that it

is not easily dressed by standard size pieces, it should by now have been possible to provide some 'made-to-measure' dressings so that the work can be done rapidly.

Subsequent changes   After the second dressing is applied, soaking through is an indication for a further complete change, which is performed as described above.

Further indications for changing the dressing are any signs suggesting that infection has supervened, i.e. pain, fever, smell.

If there are no unfavourable signs the second dressing should be left in place for 7–10 days. It is then changed again and left for 5–7 days. By this time (i.e. the third week after injury), it should be possible to tell with certainty if any of the burn is full thickness. If all the burn now appears to be partial thickness, dressings can be continued at infrequent intervals until healing is complete.

If, however, there is an obvious full thickness slough, the dressing technique is changed to one calculated to assist in removal of the slough.

Standard dressing routine   The great danger of infection of wounds during changes of dressings has been repeatedly stressed, and dressing techniques designed to minimize this danger are now part of standard nursing practice.

When burns are relatively small and involve only one surface, a 'no-touch' technique of dressing is eminently suitable. With larger and more complicated areas, however, this technique is impracticable and the dresser must be gowned and gloved as for an operation.

If an extensive circumferential burn of the trunk has to be dressed, it is often helpful to use a turning frame (e.g. Stryker frame).

When many burned patients are nursed in one ward, the performance of dressings in the open ward is highly dangerous. Colebrook and his colleagues have shown clearly that risks of infection can be much reduced by the use of a dressing room with a positive pressure (plenum) ventilating system, and this should now be considered an essential facility for all burn wards (Bourdillon and Colebrook, 1946; Colebrook, Duncan and Ross, 1948).

The majority of dressing changes can be performed without general anaesthesia, but it may be desirable to give drugs which relieve pain or diminish anxiety. These drugs may be given singly or in combination. The individual response to these drugs is variable and it may be necessary to try a number of preparations before the most suitable drug for a particular patient is found.

If pain is severe but the patient is cooperative, premixed nitrous oxide/oxygen (either 25/75 or 50/50 percentages), administered by the patient himself with a patient-demand apparatus, is excellent, and allows rapid recovery.

Of the analgesics to be given by mouth or by injection, methadone has most often been used, but pethidine, pentazocine (Fortral), phenoperidine and fentanyl have their advocates.

For sedation and tranquillizing diazepam (Valium) is excellent and can be combined with one of the analgesics mentioned above. Trimeprazine (Vallergan) is useful in children.

Suggested routine for treatment of severe burns by sulfamylon or silver sulphadiazine with minimum dressings

The first dressing should be applied as soon as the patient's general condition is satisfactory. All manipulations must be performed gently. General anaesthesia is not required but morphine should be used for sedation. The burn is cleaned with a cetrimide–chlorhexidine solution (e.g. Savlon). All loose skin is removed and blisters are snipped, the fluid is evacuated and overlying skin is removed. Sulfamylon or silver sulphadiazine is spread liberally by hand or by spatula on large sheets of gauze four layers thick. The gauze sheets are laid on the burn and smoothed into position. On the trunk the gauze sheets may be left without fixation but on the limbs it is usually convenient to hold the gauze in place by a single layer of cotton conforming bandage (Krink or Kling).

First three days   The dressings are changed daily, mopping away any discharge or old cream before a new dressing is applied.

Four to fourteen days   Once the period of maximum discharge has passed, the dressings need only be changed every other day. In an extensive burn, it may be convenient to stage the dressing changes so that, for example, opposite sides of the trunk are dressed on alternate days.

Fourteen days onwards   At 14 days, any areas of partial thickness burning will have healed or be healing. Loosened, dead tissue should be snipped away at each dressing change. With these newer antiseptics, separation of sloughs from deep partial thickness and full thickness burns is slow and if sloughs are still adherent at 21 days, late surgical excision of the sloughs should be considered (p. 85).

Bacteriology swabs
Bacteriology swabs should be taken:

(1) *On admission* – it is important to know the bacteriological state at the commencement of treatment, and failure to take a swab on admission may be regretted later.
(2) *On the third or fourth day* – in other words when the period of maximum exudation is over.
(3) *Once weekly* or more often if there is an indication.
(4) *Three days before any proposed grafting procedure*, so that the results are available before making a final decision about operation.

Infection
Some degree of bacterial contamination almost always takes place, but if all is well the burn will become dry and look undoubtedly clean and healthy. In other instances, however, clinical infection occurs, the discharge becomes wet and purulent, and there is redness at the margin of the burn.

   If haemolytic streptococcal infection occurs, the burn looks particularly angry and unhealthy. The bluish-green pus of *Ps. aeruginosa* infection is only too obvious, while *Proteus* produces large quantities of foul-smelling pus.

   Bacteria are protected by dead tissue into which antibiotics diffuse poorly and local antibiotics are of little value in the treatment of infected burns as long as dead tissue is still present. The mainstay of treatment is therefore the rapid removal of dead tissue (slough), but infection with β-haemolytic streptococci and infection with *Pseudomonas aeruginosa* require further special measures.

   The effects of invasion by β-haemolytic streptococci both locally and systemically may be serious but fortunately the organisms have remained sensitive to penicillin and other antibiotics. Systemic penicillin should be started at once and continued until wound swabs are clear. If a penicillinase-producing staphylococcus is present this may protect the streptotoccus from the penicillin and if the wound swab shows a mixed infection with streptococcus and penicillin-resistant staphylococcus, systemic treatment should be by erythromycin, cloxacillin or other antibiotics according to the bacteria sensitivity. In spite of the rather poor effect of local antibiotics, it is probably wise to use some form of local antibacterial agent not only for the sake of the infected patient, but also to minimize the chances of transferring the organisms to other patients. It is advised that NCP dressings should be used for this purpose.

If infection with *Pseudomonas aeruginosa* occurs, it is best to use frequent dressings of sulfamylon. This diffuses even into dead tissue and will often clear the organism within 7–10 days. It has the disadvantage that separation of slough is delayed and it may be necessary to carry out a surgical excision of the dead tissue (*see below*).

Local treatment of infected burns and conservative removal of slough by wet dressings

The separation of the skin slough by the development of a plane of granulation has already been described. This process is assisted by the use of a wet dressing which softens the slough. The wet dressing also has the advantage of a great initial absorptive power, which enables it to absorb the thick purulent discharge that is always present to a greater or lesser extent at this stage. The simplest dressing is the water dressing which ancients applied to all discharging wounds.

The traditional preparation for use in wet dressings is eusol (Edinburgh University Solution):

Calcium hypochlorite	1 part by weight
Boric acid	1 part by weight
Water	80 parts by weight

This is diluted to half strength with normal saline for use or to quarter strength if the patient complains of pain.

Milton (sodium hypochlorite and boric acid) has an action similar to that of eusol. Milton is cheap and easily available. Other more elegantly packed sodium hypochlorite preparations are now available (e.g. Chlorasil).

Gauze soaked in eusol and lightly wrung out is placed directly on the wound without any tulle gras or other non-adherent layer, and covered by a layer of wool or Gamgee tissue. Because the non-adherent layer has been excluded the dressing tends to stick and in order to avoid pain must often be soaked off. If the part to be dressed allows it, the most suitable method is to use a spray; in other cases a bath may be used. The bath water was traditionally of saline, but for some years only tap water has been used with no noticeable difference in results. The whole procedure of putting patients in this bath is bound to lead to some breaches an antiseptic technique, but when the dressings are adherent it leads to greatly increased comfort for the patient and is well worthwhile.

If eusol dressings are to be really effective they should never be allowed to dry out. The action of the hypochlorite is transient and eusol dressings should preferably be done three or four times a day, although this is by no means always possible. An alternative is to incorporate a number of tubes into the dressing so that the deeper layers of the dressing can be irrigated at frequent intervals.

With each change of dressing at this stage, attention should be paid to mechanical removal by forceps and scissors of any loose pieces of tissue.

Infected partial thickness burns, when the infection is brought under control, will show evidence of healing and it will then be possible to reduce the frequency of the dressings.

Particularly in deep partial thickness burns, it may still be difficult at this stage to know if epithelial elements survive, and dressings must therefore be continued until either islands of regenerating epithelium can be seen, which spread and finally coalesce, or alternatively, a uniform surface of granulation tissue forms, which indicates a full thickness burn. A smooth white layer of dermal collagen regularly spotted with red nodules of granulation tissue indicates a deep dermal burn with probably enough epithelial elements for slow healing to take place. If only a few remnants of dermal collagen are seen then few or no epithelial structures remain.

It is difficult to be sure how much good the eusol does, because its effect has never really been assessed objectively in a controlled trial. It certainly has a brief, mild, non-toxic action, and should be used if only for its fine clean antiseptic smell which encourages the patients and staff in the belief that something is being done.

In order to facilitate treatment by hypochlorite, Bunyan (1940) suggested enclosing the burn in a waterproof envelope through which hypochlorite could easily and frequently be passed. Unfortunately, because of various technical difficulties in treating the larger and more complicated burns, this method never became widely accepted. More recently Bunyan (1971, personal communication) has described the use of a new hypochlorite compound, lithium hypochlorite. This has the advantage that it is chemically more stable than either the sodium or calcium hypochlorites. Bunyan has used this in two preparations, a foam and a gel, and claims that these preparations retain their activity for eight hours or so. This would clearly very much extend the usefulness of hypochlorites, and clinical trials of these preparations are in progress.

Removal of slough by enzymes

From time to time, attempts have been made to hasten the removal of slough by the use of various enzyme preparations, acting on the assumption that the enzymes will digest any dead tissue, leaving live tissue intact – so-called 'chemical débridement'. Unfortunately, none of the preparations used so far has proved to be of practical value, but it is clear that if some chemical means could be found of removing all dead tissue, so that any area of full thickness skin loss was ready for grafting at the end of a week without the trauma of a surgical excision, this would be a great step forward. Some progress in this direction using tenderizers has recently been reported in animal experiments.

Granulations and preparation of the wound for grafting

The dressings should be continued as above until all slough has come away and the surface presents red granulations. If all has gone well the granulations will be bright or dark red, firm, flat and with little discharge and the wound is ready for grafting (*Plate 3* and *Plate 4*, *see* opposite p. 60). Unhealthy granulations are pale, friable, raised, oedematous and hypertrophic looking and often associated with a copious discharge of pus.

The chance of grafts taking depends largely on the character of the granulations, and with a little practice the healthy granulations on which grafts take with certainty can instantly be recognized. Under these circumstances bacteriological examination is little more than a formality.

If the granulations are unhealthy, however, every effort should be made to improve them by treatment before applying grafts. The types or organisms present and their antibiotic sensitivity should be determined. If β-haemolytic streptococci are present treatment should be by local and systemic penicillin, and grafting should not be performed until the organisms have been cleared.

If staphylococci are the main organisms present it is difficult to decide if antibiotics should be used. If much pus is present NPC cream applied daily may be effective.

If the granulations are oedematous an ointment containing terramycin and hydrocortisone (Terracortryl) should be tried.

If *Pseudomonas aeruginosa* is present then daily dressings of sulfamylon should be applied. It is also important with Gram-negative infections to get rid of dead tissue and every opportunity at dressing changes should be taken to remove dead tissue by snipping it away with scissors. *Proteus vulgaris* infection may be treated by antibiotics of the polymyxin, bacitracin and neomycin group, although the results are often disappointing and skin grafting will usually have to be undertaken with the organisms still present. Success can still be obtained in wounds infected with *Proteus* or *Pseudomonas*, if the grafts are dressed early or exposed.

Systemic antibiotics

The administration of antibiotics in conventional doses (e.g. 250 mg of penicillin 8-hourly) does not prevent bacterial colonization of the burn and examination of the burn exudate in patients so treated shows little or no antibiotic. However if much larger doses are given (e.g. 1.0 g of penicillin 4-hourly) then useful levels of antibiotics can be detected in the exudate.

Systemic antibiotics are of undoubted value in the treatment of bacterial invasion of the soft tissues and of the blood stream but it is disappointing to find how often antibiotics fail to prevent bacterial invasion when administered prophylactically.

Initial period
Patients with burns of less than 10 per cent of the body surface area are not in great danger from infection and routine systemic antibiotics need not be given. With more extensive burns systemic penicillin should be given by injection (not by mouth) for the first few days to make certain that the wound presents an unfavourable climate for the β-haemolytic streptococcus, which is still a danger to burns patients because of its destructive effects on surviving epithelium. It is recommended that systemic penicillin in high dosage (1 mega-unit 4-hourly) be given from the outset, until a satisfactory crust has formed if the patient is being treated by exposure, or until a second dressing has been done with a patient treated by dressings.

Later period
This important subject, including treatment of invasive sepsis and septicaemia, is considered in Chapter 4 (pp. 105–109).

Grafting

When the sloughs have separated and healthy granulations have been obtained, skin grafts should be applied to obtain epithelialization of the wound in all cases where the raw areas are more than 2.5 cm (1 inch) wide.

The skin grafts to be used are thin split skin (Thiersch) grafts cut from any suitable uninjured part of the body.

The operation is performed in the operating theatre under a general anaesthetic.

Instrumentarium

The instruments available are:

(1) Blair knife – the simplest instrument, being a straight flat blade. The use of this instrument requires practice, but it is possible to cut excellent thin grafts. A convex donor site is essential.
(2) Humby knife – this knife, which has a roller, is an excellent instrument, and undoubtedly the best for the surgeon who cuts grafts relatively infrequently. The modern versions with replaceable blades (Bodenham and Braithwaite) are particularly useful.
(3) Electric dermatone – this instrument cuts good grafts rapidly and is of great value in extensive burns where speed is essential. The instrument developed by Davis of Cape Town is a great advance on previous models.
(4) Padgett dermatome – an instrument which is most useful for cutting single thick grafts, but is not particularly suitable for multiple thin grafts in burned patients. However, it may sometimes be used when only the trunk is available as a donor site, because it is the only instrument which will cut satisfactorily from a concave area, as on the abdomen.
(5) Reese dermatone – is more suitable for thin grafts than the Padgett dermatone, but is not often available in this country.

Donor sites and cutting of graft

The donor sites in order of ease and preference are as follows:

   (1) Thigh.
   (2) Lower legs.
   (3) Arm.
   (4) Trunk.

Grafts can be cut satisfactorily from the limbs by a Blair or Humby knife or the electric dermatome.

For the trunk the electric dermatome is most generally employed, but sometimes a knife can be used and occasionally the Padgett dermatome is useful.

The grafts are cut as thin as possible. Theoretically, they should be cut as a clean procedure before exposing or handling the granulating area. In practice this is not obligatory and donor sites rarely become infected.

After removal of grafts the donor sites are dressed with tulle gras, gauze, wool and bandage. (*See Figure 3.6.*)

Treatment of the recipient area

The granulations are wiped with a swab moistened with saline to remove fibrin debris. If a white network of dermal fibres is present this may be removed by firm wiping with gauze, but care should be taken to avoid making the surface bleed.

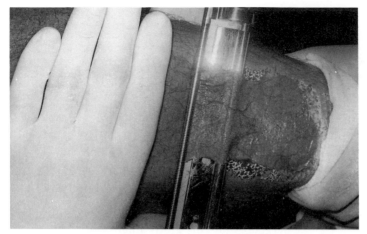

(a)

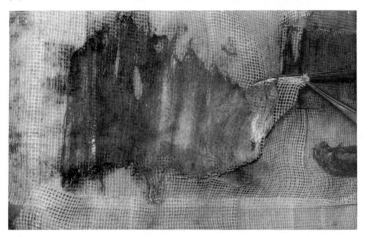

(b)

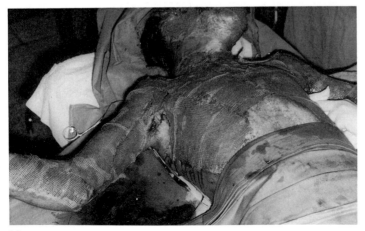

(c)

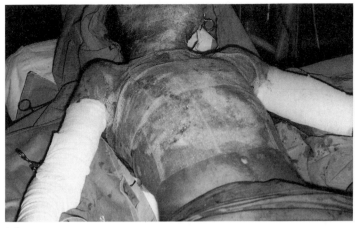

(d)

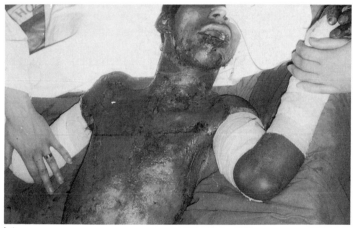

(e)

Figure 3.6 (a) A sheet of skin is cut with a Braithwaite knife. (b) The skin is backed with Jelonet for ease of handling. (c) Grafts applied to the granulating areas. (d) A large sheet of Jelonet is applied overall, and the area exposed without further cover. (e) Full take of skin after 6 days

Handling of the graft

To facilitate ease of handling the grafts are spread, raw surface upwards, on tulle gras which is then cut round the margin of the grafts. The grafts are then cut into suitable shapes and sizes.

As soon as the grafts have been spread and cut they are applied to the raw area. If the granulations are healthy, the grafts may be applied in large strips or patches, but it is easy to waste time by trying to make pieces fit and it is usually time saving to cut the grafts into fairly large pieces.

If there is considerable infection of the granulations, there is much to be said for the time-honoured method of applying the grafts in 'postage stamp' size (e.g. 2.5×5 cm) or in long narrow strips. The grafts should be laid edge to edge. Any excess of skin graft remaining at the end of the operation, may be stored in the refrigerator (*see* p. 84), for use at a later date to patch up any areas where grafts have failed to take.

After-treatment of grafts
The grafts may be treated by dressings or by exposure.

Dressings   The grafts are covered by a layer of tulle gras applied in large sheets which fix the grafts in position and prevent them slipping around while the outer dressings are applied.

The dressing is completed by layers of gauze, wool and bandages in the usual way.

Change of dressings   The time of first change of dressings depends on the amount of infection and the nature of the organisms present.

If the granulations are firm and healthy with little pus the dressing may be left for a week. However, if much pus is being formed the dressing must be changed earlier and, if Gram-negative organisms are present, then the dressings must be changed at two days and frequently thereafter.

To prevent pulling off the grafts, an inner layer of tulle gras should be applied until 10 days after grafting, when any graft which has taken will be stable. Any loose bits of graft which are overlapping or have not taken are snipped off at each dressing.

If there is much infection, eusol dressings should be applied over tulle gras until any surviving grafts are stable, when the tulle gras can be omitted.

As soon as the grafts are becoming stable (i.e. about 10 days), it is as well to change over to frequent eusol dressing for a short period. This helps to get rid of any odd bits of graft which have not taken and cleans up the wound so as to facilitate final healing by outgrowth of skin cells to bridge the small gaps between the grafts.

Treatment of grafts by exposure
For many years it was generally believed that it was necessary to apply pressure to a graft if it was to take. It is now known that a graft will take satisfactorily as long as it is not mechanically displaced or lifted off its bed by haematoma or pus formation. Grafting without dressings is particularly suitable for:

(1) *Heavily infected areas*, particularly when Gram-negative organisms are present. These organisms thrive in the dark, moist and warm conditions under a dressing and will often float the grafts off because of the volume of pus they produce. Under the conditions of exposure (*Figure 3.7*), however, the activity of these organisms is diminished and grafts have a much better chance of survival.

(2) *Areas which cannot be satisfactorily immobilized under dressings* – in some regions, e.g. the neck, the part may very easily move inside the relatively fixed mass of dressings, and grafts will then be rubbed off. If the grafts are simply laid on, however, they immediately adhere and can be seen to move with their underlying bed during movements of the head or during swallowing.

The trunk and buttocks are other areas which are suitable for grafting without dressings.

For reasons of convenience and also on account of discharge it is often advisable to treat the grafts initially by exposure and then, on the fourth day, by which time a fair degree of adherence will have occurred, to change over to treatment by dressings.

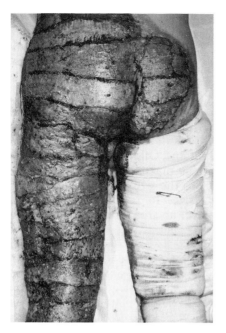

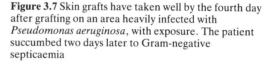

Figure 3.7 Skin grafts have taken well by the fourth day after grafting on an area heavily infected with *Pseudomonas aeruginosa*, with exposure. The patient succumbed two days later to Gram-negative septicaemia

Delayed application of grafts

Some areas are difficult to dress satisfactorily in an anaesthetized patient and there is a danger that the grafts may be displaced during the recovery from anaesthesia. This is likely to occur in burns of the neck and trunk and particularly in large and heavy patients. Under these circumstances, it is a good practice to cut the grafts, store them in a refrigerator for one to two days until the patient is conscious and cooperative, and then apply the grafts in the dressing room or in the patient's bed without further anaesthesia. Delayed application of grafts is also desirable when an excision has been performed and there is oozing of blood from the raw area which cannot be adequately controlled.

Graft failures

Because of infection some of the grafts may fail to take. If this occurs, every attempt must be made by suitable dressings to clean up the granulations and, if the loss of grafts has been considerble, then further grafting should be carried out.

Later stage

In extensive burns, and particularly when infection has caused difficulty in getting grafts to take, a state will be reached when the burned area is covered by more or less stable grafts with intervening granulating areas which are not large enough to warrant grafting. Final healing under these conditions may be very slow and may try the patience of doctors, nurses and patient. The changes may be rung on different dressings and there is no general rule for deciding which one may be suitable in a particular case. When the raw areas are small it is sometimes a good thing to paint them with mercurochrome in spirit, forming a dry scab under which epithelialization can become complete.

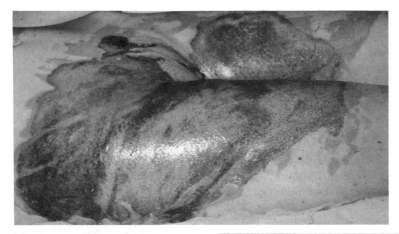

(a)

(b)

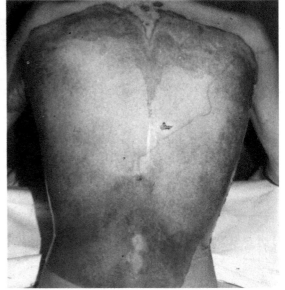

Plate 2 Comparison of the appearance of burns of different depths. (*a*) Superficial burn: the surface is pink and looks moist. (*b*) Deep dermal burn: this whitish appearance is typical of deep dermal involvement (the more superficial areas can be seen around the periphery). (*c*) Deep burn: the dry dark-brown colour, with the presence of thrombosed vessels evident in the eschar, is characteristic of a deep burn

(c)

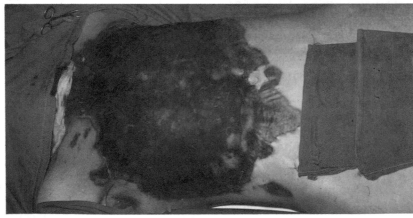

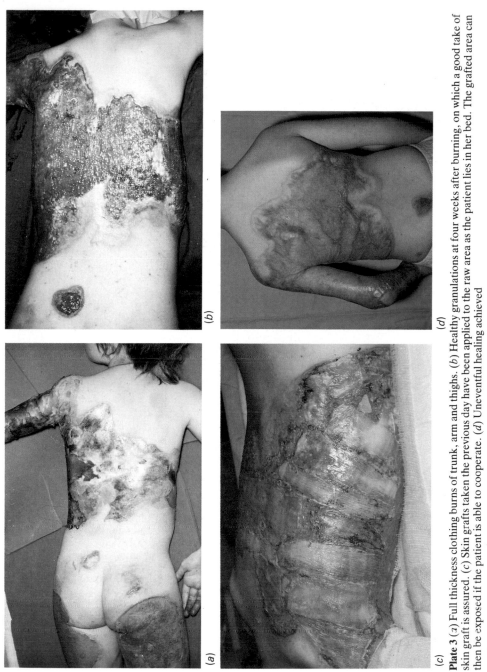

Plate 3 (*a*) Full thickness clothing burns of trunk, arm and thighs. (*b*) Healthy granulations at four weeks after burning, on which a good take of skin graft is assured. (*c*) Skin grafts taken the previous day have been applied to the raw area as the patient lies in her bed. The grafted area can then be exposed if the patient is able to cooperate. (*d*) Uneventful healing achieved

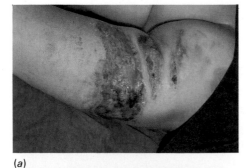

(a)

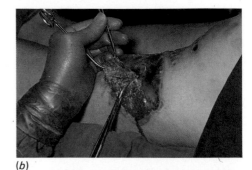

(b)

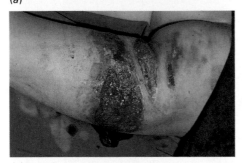

(c)

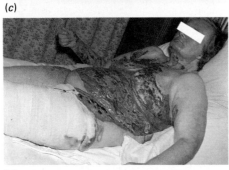

(d)

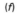

(e)

(f)

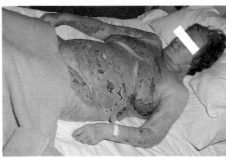

(g)

Plate 4 (*a*) Small full-thickness burns from leaking hot water bottle. (*b*) Surgical excision of slough on the fourth day after burning is simple for burns of this size. (*c*) A satisfactory surface which will accept skin grafts is produced. (*d*) The area is healed 10 days after burning: a great deal of time can be saved by early surgery in suitable cases. (*e*) Heavy elderly patient after five weeks of dressings for a full thickness burn of the trunk. Parts of the burned area have granulated well, firmly adherent slough remains in some places. (*f*) Closure of the major part of the wound by skin grafting has markedly improved the patient's general condition. Healthy granulations are now present where previously slough had been adherent. (*g*) Good healing by accepting two moderately sized operations in preference to one major and more dangerous operation

(Cochrane, 1968). This technique is not part of normal clinical practice, and will not have much application for autograft skin. It does, however, have considerable application for skin homografts (*see below*).

Note: if small pieces of skin are left over following a grafting operation, and it is desirable to avoid a further anaesthetic, the pieces can very conveniently be stored on the donor site, as described by Shepard (1972).

Late excision of a slough

The programme which has been outlined, i.e. conservative treatment to prevent infection, wet dressings to expedite removal of slough, and grafting, is an orthodox and well-tried routine which has given good results in many cases and is suitable for most severe burns.

In some cases, however, usually those which have been treated by dressings and in whom infection has been well controlled, the position may arise that between the fourteenth and twenty-first day the area of partial thickness burning has healed, leaving a well-demarcated area of obvious full thickness slough which is still firmly adherent to the underlying tissues. Under these conditions it is possible to expedite matters by a surgical slough excision under anaesthesia.

The sloughs are removed by dissection with scissors in the plane of natural separation, which at this stage can be easily found. If the raw surface is healthy when the slough has been removed, then grafts may be cut and applied immediately, but if the surface looks unhealthy, eusol dressings should be applied and continued until healthy granulations are obtained and before grafting is attempted.

The bleeding during slough excision is moderate and soon stops, and grafts take well. Blood transfusion is usually required. Under present conditions, treatment of burns by late slough excision and grafting is the ideal to be aimed for in most serious burns.

The indications for slough excision are more obvious when dressings have been used than when the burn has been exposed. Separation of crust from areas of deep partial thickness burn treated by exposure may be slow and it is easy to remove viable epithelial cells by performing slough excision too early.

If some degree of infection has already developed and the slough is beginning to come away, surgical slough excision does not greatly accelerate matters and is probably better not done.

Evans (1953) uses a Humby knife or electric dermatome with the gap set wide open for the excision and at this stage the blade tends to follow the natural plane of separation.

Early excision and grafting

The methods of treatment which have been described so far are orthodox methods suitable for many severe burns in which the presence or extent of whole thickness burning is indefinite when the patient is first seen. In a minority of patients, however, it is possible to shorten the duration of the illness and to aim for improved final results by surgical excision of dead skin and grafting at an early stage. Two different types of surgical technique must be considered:

(1) Scalpel excision.
(2) Tangential excision by means of a skin grafting knife.

The application of these techniques to three different types of burns is discussed below:

(1) Undoubted full thickness burns with clearly defined edges up to 10 per cent surface area.
(2) Moderately extensive burns typically of deep partial thickness depth but possibly with some full thickness patches.
(3) Extensive life-threatening burns with deep partial thickness and full thickness depth.

Full thickness burns with clearly defined edges – up to 10 per cent surface area

In a small group of patients there is, on first examination, an obviously full thickness burn with clearly defined edges. This is typically found in burns sustained by direct contact, e.g. with a hot radiator or coal fire, but is also seen occasionally in flame burns and in some chemical injuries. The ideal treatment for this type of burn is surgical excision of the dead skin and grafting at the earliest opportunity. Excision of up to 5 per cent surface area presents few problems and gives excellent results (*see Plate 4a, b,* opposite p. 60). In experienced hands excisions of burns up to 10 per cent are feasible. The operation is performed by sharp dissection with a scalpel and is associated with brisk haemorrhage. An excision of 10 per cent surface area may cause blood loss equivalent to half the patient's blood volume and this loss must of course be made good by simultaneous transfusion (Muir and Grummitt, 1957). If limbs are involved, use should be made of high elevation or tourniquets to reduce blood loss and, in burns of the face and head, such as may be sustained by epileptics, hypotensive drugs are of value. If the area to be excised is small and speed is not essential, the best cosmetic result may be obtained by performing the excision at the most superficial layer of viable tissue. When extensive areas are involved, however, we prefer to excise all skin and fat, since in most parts of the body a good plane is found immediately superficial to the deep fascia. At this level, the excision can be expeditious, bleeding points are few and easily controlled and the raw surface is excellent for the reception of grafts. An excision of 10 per cent area will stretch the resources of most operating teams. Even larger excisions of 20 per cent or more have been carried out in special centres. These operations are not part of standard practice, but are further considered below.

Time of excision
If the *total* area of burn is 10 per cent or less the operation can safely be performed at the earliest convenient time – on the first day if possible.

In burns greater than this size, continued plasma loss from areas of partial thickness burn or deeper unexcised tissues, may cause difficulties if operation is performed during the first two days and, in these cases, therefore, it is our practice to carry the patient through the shock period with the usual management and then to perform the excision on the third, fourth or fifth day.

At this time the patient is usually in good condition and the delay is valuable in allowing the organization of staff and procuring the blood which is so vital.

Moderately extensive deep partial thickness burns possibly with some areas of full thickness loss

As has mentioned, these burns characteristically heal spontaneously but with the formation of hypertrophic scars.

It has been explained that the important histological factor of the deep partial thickness burn is that the fat 'domes' are penetrated and they are the sites of granulation tissue reaction. This can be well seen at the stage of separation of slough from a deep partial thickness burn when rounded nodules of granulation tissue can be seen against a white background of surviving dermis. Typically each nodule of granulation tissue contains a hair root. From this stage on the outcome depends on a race between the evolving granulation tissue and the regenerating epithelium. In a few cases, epithelialization proceeds rapidly and this seems to cut short the granulation reaction so that hypertrophy of the scar does not occur.

In the majority of cases, however, the balance is tipped in favour of the granulation reaction. The epithelial remnants appear to be trapped in the bases of the granulations and, by the time the regenerating epithelial cells reach the surface, the granulation reaction is well established and in some way self-perpetuating so that, even when epithelialization is complete, the condition evolves into a hypertrophic scar.

In order to avoid this sequence of events, two techniques have been evolved:

(1) Early tangential evasion and overgrafting.
(2) Late abrasion of granulations with or without grafting.

Early tangential excision and overgrafting
This technique is suitable for burns of suspected deep partial thickness or mixed deep partial and full thickness burns and has been developed particularly by Janzekovic (1968) of Yugoslavia.

The proponents of this technique make the point that operation is to some extent diagnostic, that superficial partial thickness burns will be recognized immediately on shaving and need not be covered by grafts, and that conversely only those burns which really need grafting will be so treated.

Operation is performed three days after burning so that any predetermined and therefore inevitable progression of the burn depth will have taken place and the burn is still sterile.

Progressive layers of skin are shaved off the burned area using a skin grafting knife. The appearance of bleeding spots indicates that shaving is deep enough. If a large number of small bleeding points appear at a very superficial level the burn is a superficial partial thickness burn and skin grafting is not necessary.

If shaving has to be deeper and exposes a smaller number of freely bleeding points then the burn is of deep partial thickness depth and the raw area should be covered by skin grafts (*Figure 3.8*).

Many surgeons consider that by this method the maximum amount of dermal collagen is saved and that this adds to the quality of the finally healed skin.

Other workers, however, have had reservations about this treatment and have been concerned that, if Janzekovic's criteria are followed, some patients will have unnecessary operations.

Page and Barclay (1981) reported on 72 children with scalds, using the criteria advised by Jackson and Stone (1972) for selecting patients suitable for early excision and grafting. They divided the children into two groups:

(i) Thirty-four patients whose scalds were considered to be of superficial partial thickness depth and who were expected to heal without scarring.
(ii) Thirty-eight patients who were expected to heal with scarring, i.e. who were thought to have areas of deep partial thickness burns.

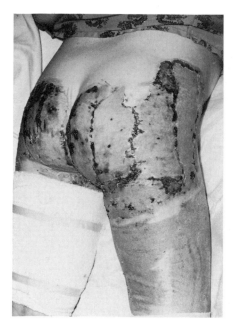

Figure 3.8 Satisfactory healing of deep dermal burns of buttocks 10 days after treatment by tangential excision and grafting on the third day after burning

The patients were then all treated conservatively. Of the 34 patients who were expected to have no scarring, 11 showed scars when healed and of the 38 who were all expected to have scars 13 healed without scars. In other words, if the usual criteria are used, one in three children will have an unnecessary operation.

However, the lack of any test for depth of injury in young children, other than careful inspection of the surface of the burn (because the pinprick test (*see* p. 62) is usually impracticable) should not discourage the surgeon from employing tangential excision (*Figure 3.9*) and skin grafting when he is reasonably certain that the injury has damaged the deep dermis and will be accompanied by slow healing with scarring in the absence of early surgery. This particularly applies to burns of the dorsum of the hand in adults (for whom the pinprick test is usually very informative), where successful tangential excision and grafting on the third day will produce a completely healed hand by the tenth day (*see* Chapter 5, p. 125). This represents a very great saving of hospital time and patient discomfort, and the quality of skin cover is usually outstandingly good, with corresponding minimization of embarrassing scarring in a very prominent area.

Mahler and Hirshowitz (1975), describing their experience of treatment of 69 hands in three weeks by tangential excision, following the Yom Kippur War (1973), were in no doubt of its value in the mass casualty situation also. 'Early tangential excision of deep burns has many advantages, particularly in hands; the oedema and infection which accompany spontaneous desloughing are eliminated; pain is abolished; there is no need for lengthy splintage or fixation; hospital stay is reduced to days rather than weeks.'

This opinion is fully concurred with by the authors. Following the football stand fire at Bradford (1985), 55 hands were dealt with by tangential excision and grafting in a period of three days, and primary healing obtained in more than 90 per cent of cases. If, in a mass casualty situation, logistics permit aggressive treatment of burned hands, this should have a high priority (*see* Chapter 9, p. 170).

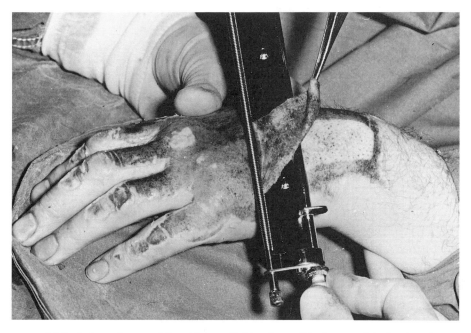

Figure 3.9 Technique of tangential excision applied to a burn of the dorsum of the hand, under tourniquet

Late abrasion of granulations with or without skin grafting

An additional factor which must be taken into consideration is that tangential excision and grafting requires large resources in terms of personnel and operating time. To avoid the risk of operating on burns which will heal rapidly, and also to make skin grafting operations easier to fit into fixed operating schedules, an alternative procedure is suggested, as follows (Holmes and Rayner, 1984):

> The patient is treated conservatively for 2–3 weeks until the sloughs have separated. If the appearance of deep dermal burning is seen, operation is arranged.
>
> The granulations are removed by light surgical abrasion. If the residual dermis forms a good firm layer nothing further is done and most of these cases progress to rapid epithelialization with no subsequent hypertrophic scar formation.
>
> It seems as if the removal of the granulations releases the epithelial elements which now produce rapid epithelial cover which, in its turn, inhibits the formation of further granulations.
>
> If the abrasion exposes an incomplete ragged layer of dermis, it is unlikely that enough epithelial elements remain to be of value and the raw area is therefore covered by skin grafts – either in sheets or a mesh whichever seems appropriate.

Excision of burns on a life-saving measure

Of the value of early excision of burns in relieving the period of pain and misery, shortening the time during which the patient is at risk of infection and improving healing there can be no doubt. The value of early excision of extensive burns in improving the chances of survival is less certain, and the choice between a conservative type of regimen under good circumstances and an extensive early operation for a life-threatening burn is not clearcut.

Opinion has swung more in favour of early operation because of certain recent improvements in techniques and has been highlighted by the unprecedent results produced by Chinese surgeons in saving patients with deep burns of over 90 per cent of the body surface who would previously have had no hope of survival.

The technical improvements are in the fields of:

Antibiotics.
Anaesthetic techniques.
Instrumentation for taking grafts and expanding grafts.
Use of homo- and xenografts.

The contribution of surgery is in achieving the quickest skin cover with minimal donor area for providing grafts. This has been achieved in two ways:

(1) By meshing and marked expansion of the grafts even in the proportions of 1:9 and then covering the whole area with allografts or xenografts.
(2) The Chinese method which consists in covering the whole of the excised area with sheets of allograft which are stitched together. A few days later the allografts are perforated at regular intervals, the perforations are allowed to gape and the gaps are filled by tiny autografts. This may involve a simple but very time-consuming surgical procedure to be carried out every day for weeks or even months on end.

Repeated use of donor sites
If the available donor areas are small in relation to the area to be grafted, it may be necessary to use the same donor area on two or more occasions. To enable this to be done the grafts must be cut as thin as possible. Usually 2–3 weeks will elapse before grafts can be cut from the same site again.

Priorities

If sufficient grafts are not available to cover the whole area at one sitting how should they be disposed? A number of factors must be taken into account, some of them contradictory.

Coverage can be increased by using mesh grafts for all sites except the face and hands where both function and appearance are better if sheet grafts are used.

Three sites have priority so far as skin cover is concerned:

(1) The eyelids.
(2) The hands.
(3) The neck.

The eyelids have over-riding priority at all times but the other sites may have to take second place if it is necessary to cover as much area as possible in a life-threatening situation. Under these circumstances it may not be reasonable to spend the time which is necessary to apply skin grafts to the raw surfaces of the hands.

(4) Good healthy granulating areas should receive preference over areas with poor granulations, on which grafts have a poor chance of taking.

(5) Areas which are mechanically easier to graft, e.g. limbs, should receive preference over areas where graft may be rubbed off, e.g. loins.
(6) In circumferential burns it is preferable to graft only one surface (i.e. anterior or posterior) of the body at a time to give grafts the best chance of taking.
(7) It is sometimes a good thing from the nursing point of view to concentrate grafts in one area, i.e. one limb, so as to get it healed in order to facilitate handling, and reduce the number of areas which have to be dressed.
(8) If a larger raw area exists than can be covered by sheet grafts then the grafts should be meshed.

Homografts (allografts) and heterografts (xenografts)

The grafts ordinarily used for the resurfacing of burned areas are of course autografts, i.e. taken from the uninjured parts of the patient's body. Homografts (allografts), i.e. grafts taken from another person, may be used under certain circumstances to give temporary cover. With the exception of grafts taken from identical twins, they are cast off after three to four weeks due to the development of antibodies. In the early stages, however, they take well and are indistinguishable from autografts. Improved methods of preventing infection have reduced the number of cases in which homografting is necessary. Homografts have been used in many different ways, but at the present moment, their usefulness is proven only in a few special circumstances:

(1) As the sole cover for a granulating area, if the patient is so ill that an operation to remove autografts cannot be undertaken. This temporary closure of the burned area may well allow the patient to recover, and permit autografting later.
(2) To complete the cover of an extensive granulating area when insufficient autografts are available, and it is felt that leaving the area raw would put the patient seriously at risk.
(3) In combination with small areas of autografts when extensive burns are excised as a life-saving procedure (*see below*).

Source and type of homografts

Donated skin
If it is known some days in advance that homografts will be necessary, small amounts of extra skin may be taken from other patients requiring skin grafting and stored in the refrigerator at +4°C or −4°C as described above. If skin is needed at short notice, then skin donors must be found among healthy relatives of the patient, or volunteers called for from patients having general anaesthesia for other operations. It is, of course, imperative that the donor should be healthy and the nature of their operation such that their recovery will not be jeopardized by the taking of the grafts. It is a happy commentary on human nature that we have never failed to find willing volunteers for this procedure.

Cadaver skin
Some centres where large numbers of serious burns are treated have established skin banks of cadaver skin. Recent work at East Grinstead (Hackett and Batchelor, 1971) using tissue typing has shown that the survival of homografts is prolonged if the tissue types of the donor and recipient are close. The skin is most useful if it is preserved in a live state and it is, therefore, dehydrated with glycerol and stored in

a deep freeze, having previously been tissue typed. When a burned patient requires homograft skin, his tissue type is compared with the skin available in the bank and the most suitable type is selected.

Freeze-dried (lyophilized) skin
This is usually again cadaver skin, first frozen and then completely dried. It is non-viable, but has the advantage that it can be stored indefinitely and also that when it is applied it does not provoke the development of antibodies. It is useful as a temporary cover when suitable live homograft skin is not available.

Heterografts (xenografts)

Grafts from animals, usually pigs and calves, have been used in experimental and clinical trials, but their value is still uncertain.

If all goes well epithelium spreads out from the autografts and the allografts are rejected, but in addition the Chinese claim that only the epithelium of the allografts is cast off and that the (non-cellular) dermis is overgrown by the patient's epithelium and incorporated in a healed skin of much better quality than could be achieved by the autografts alone.

It is difficult at the moment to know how widely it will be possible to apply these techniques. In the past it has seemed that the trauma of the burn itself has inhibited both the healing reaction and the resistance to infection and that the extra trauma of operation has exacerbated these effects and the patient has died some days later from uncontrolled septicaemia and with no sign of healing reaction in the wound.

Summary

Inspect burn on admission and try to determine depth.

(1) *Burn is obviously superficial*
> Treat conservatively.
>
> *Dress –* discrete burn of limb or trunk which can be completely and adequately dressed.
>
> *Expose –* burn of face, perineum, single surface burn of trunk and any others which cannot be completely dressed.

(2) *Burn is obviously deep and less than 10 per cent area*
> Consider early excision and grafting (possibly up to 20 per cent in special centres). Particularly useful in deep localized burns of face and head in epileptics.

(3) *Burn is of doubtful depth*
> *Either* (*a*) Treat conservatively for 14–21 days as in (1) above.
>
> At 14–21 days if full thickness burn is clearly demarcated, consider late excision and grafting.
>
> Otherwise change over to frequent eusol dressings and graft granulating area when healthy.
>
> (*b*) Consider early tangential excision of as much deep partial thickness area as can be resurfaced by autografts.

(4) *Burn is deep, but more than 10 per cent*
> Treat as for (3*a*), unless circumstances are particularly favourable for scalpel excision up to the limits of concurrent autografting.

References

BARCLAY, T. L. (1970) *ChM Thesis*. University of Edinburgh

BARCLAY, T. L. (1971) Faecal *Pseudomonas aeruginosa* in patients with burns. In *Transactions of Fifth International Congress of Plastic and Reconstructive Surgery*. p. 843. Sydney: Butterworths

BARCLAY, T. L. and DEXTER, F. (1968) Infection and cross-infection in a new Burns Centre. *British Journal of Surgery*, **55**, 197

BOURDILLON, R. B. and COLEBROOK, L. (1946) Air hygiene in dressing rooms for burns or major wounds. *Lancet*, **i**, 561, 601

BUNYAN, J. (1940) Envelope method of treating burns. *British Medical Journal*, **2**, 680

CASON, J. S. and LOWBURY, E. J. L. (1960) Prophylactic chemotherapy for burns. *Lancet*, **ii**, 501

COCHRANE, T. (1968) The low temperature storage of skin: a preliminary report. *British Journal of Plastic Surgery*, **21**, 118

COLEBROOK, L. (1950) *A New Approach to the Treatment of Burns and Scalds*. London: Fine Technical Publications

COLEBROOK, L., CLARK, A. M., GIBSON, T. and TODD, J. P. (1945) Studies of burns and scalds. *Special Report Series of the Medical Research Council (London)*, No. 249

COLEBROOK, L., DUNCAN, J. M. and ROSS, W. P. D. (1948) The control of infection in burns. *Lancet*, **i**, 893

CRUICKSHANK, R. (1935) The bacterial infection of burns. *Journal of Pathology and Bacteriology*, **41**, 367

DAVIS, J. H., ARTZ, C. P., REISS, E. and AMSPACHER, W. H. (1953) Practical technics in the case of the burn patient. *American Journal of Surgery*, **86**, 713

DEPARTMENT OF HEALTH, SCOTLAND (1942) Emergency Medical Services Memorandum 8. *Hospital Treatment of Burns*. Edinburgh: HMSO

EVANS, A. J. (1953) The early treatment of burns at a regional plastic centre. *British Journal of Plastic Surgery*, **5**, 263

EVANS, A. J. (1957) Experiences of a burns unit – review of 520 cases. *British Medical Journal*, **2**, 547

FOX, C. L., Jr (1968) Silver sulphadiazine – a new topical therapy for pseudomonas infection in burns. *Archives of Surgery*, **96**(2), 184

GAMGEE, S. (1876). The treatment of wounds. *Lancet*, **ii**, 885

HACKETT, M. E. and BATCHELOR, J. R. (1971) The HL-A system and its importance for skin grafting in burned patients. In *Research in Burns. Transactions of the Third Congress on Research in Burns*, Prague, 1970. Bern: Hans Huber

HOLMES, J. D. and RAYNER, C. R. W. (1984) The technique of late dermabrasion for deep dermal burns. *Burns*, **10**, 347

JACKSON, D. McG. (1953) The diagnosis of the depth of burning. *British Journal of Surgery*, **40**, 588

JACKSON, D. McG. (1969) Second thoughts on the burn wound. *Journal of Trauma*, **9**, 839

JACKSON, D. McG., LOWBURY, E. J. L. and TOPLEY, E. (1951) *Pseudomonas pyocyanea* in burns. *Lancet*, **ii**, 137

JACKSON, D. McG. and STONE, P. A. (1972) Tangential excision and grafting of burns – the method and a report on 50 consecutive cases. *British Journal of Pharmacological Science*, **27**, 417

JANZEKOVIC, Z. (1968) Consistent application of generally adopted surgical principles in the treatment of the burn wound. In *Present Clinical Aspects of Burns*. Ed. M. Derganc. Published by the Organising Committee of the 3rd Yugoslav Congress of Plastic and Maxillo-Facial Surgery, Maribor, Yugoslavia

LANZ, O. (1908) *Zentralblatt für Cherurgie*, **35**, 3. Die transplantation betreffend

LINDBERG, R., MONCRIEF, J. A., SWITZER, W. E., ODDER, S. E. and MILLS, W. (1965) The successful control of burn wound sepsis. *Journal of Trauma*, **6**, 407

LISTER, J. (1867) On a new method of treating compound fracture, abscess, etc. *Lancet*, **i**, 326, 357, 387, 507; **ii**, 95

LISTER, J. (1907) Note on the double cyanide of mercury and zinc as an antiseptic dressing. *British Medical Journal*, **1**, 795

LOWBURY, E. J. L. (1960) Infection of burns. *British Medical Journal*, **1**, 194

LOWBURY, E. J. L. and HOOD, A. M. (1952) A disinfectant barrier in dressings applied to burns. *Lancet*, **i**, 899

LOWBURY, E. J. L., KIDSON, A., LILLY, H. A., AYLIFFE, G. A. J. and JONES, R. J. (1969) Carbenicillin resistance of *Ps. aeruginosa*. *Lancet*, **ii**, 448, 473

MAHLER, D. and HIRSHOWITZ, B. (1975) Tangential excision and grafting for burns of the hand. *British Journal of Plastic Surgery,* **28,** 189–192

MOYER, C. A., BRENTANO, L., CRAVENS, D. L., MARGRAF, H. W. and MONAFO, W. W., Jr (1965) Treatment of large human burns with 0.5 per cent silver nitrate solution. *Archives of Surgery,* **90,** 812

MUIR, I. F. K. and GRUMMITT, M. J. (1957) Early excision of burns with particular reference to blood replacement. In *Transactions of the International Society of Plastic Surgeons* (1st Congress 1955), p. 98. Baltimore: Williams and Wilkins

MUIR, I. F. K., OWEN, D. and MURPHY, J. (1969) Sulfamylon acetate in the treatment of *Pseudomonas pyocyanea* infection of burns. *British Journal of Plastic Surgery,* **22,** 201

MUIR, I. F. K. and STRANC, M. F. (1966) The micro-cimate of the burn surface. In *Research in Burns. Transactions of the Second International Congress on Research in Burnsx,* Edinburgh, 1965, p. 586. Edinburgh: Livingstone

PAGE, R. E. and BARCLAY, T. L. (1981) Correlation of scald depth and hypertrophic scar formation. *Burns,* **7,** 173

SANDERS, R., SCALES, J. T. and MUIR, I. F. K. (1970) Levitation in the treatment of large area burns. *Lancet,* **ii,** 677

SCALES, J. T., HOPKINS, L. A., BLOCH, M., TOWERS, A. G. and MUIR, I. F. K. (1967) Levitation in the treatment of large area burns. *Lancet,* **i,** 1235

SHARPE, D. T., ROBERTS, A. H. N., BARCLAY, T. L., DICKSON, W. A., SETTLE, J. A. D., CROCKETT, D. J. *et al.* (1985) Treatment of burns casualties after fire at Bradford City Football Ground (1985), *British Medical Journal,* **291,** 945–949

SHEPARD, G. H. (1972) The storage of split-skin grafts on donor sites. *Plastic Reconstructive Surgery,* **49,** 115

SYME, J. (1837) *The Principles of Surgery,* 2nd edn. Edinburgh: John Stark

TANNER, J. C., VANDEPUT, J. and OLLEY, J. F. (1964) The mesh skin graft. *Plastic and Reconstructive Surgery,* **34,** 287

WALLACE, A. B. (1949) Treatment of burns; a return to basic principles. *British Journal of Plastic Surgery,* **1,** 232

WALLACE, A. B. (1951) The exposure treatment of burns. *Lancet,* **i,** 501

WALLACE, A. B. (1952) Burns: some experiences in local care. *British Journal of Plastic Surgery,* **4,** 224

Chapter 4

General care of patients with burns and scalds

If a patient with an extensive burn is to be kept in good shape to withstand his prolonged illness, with probably one or more severe operations, his general condition must be carefully attended to.

General nursing precautions

Every effort should be made to prevent bacterial contamination of the burned surface, since infection and fatal septicaemia are the main dangers to patients with large burns who have survived the shock period.

Cleansing the hands

Careful and thorough hand hygiene is of paramount importance in preventing the transmission of infection to or from the burns patient. Consequently, the patient should never be handled without prior hand cleansing and, after the patient or his bedclothes have been handled, the hands and forearms must be cleansed again. Relatively casual hand washing commonly leaves the tips of the fingers and much of the thumbs hardly cleansed at all (Taylor, 1978) and thorough hand cleansing requires systematic attention to all parts of the hands. Warm water and soap are the obvious choice to cleanse soiled hands, followed, after the final water rinse, by the use of an alcoholic solution of chlorhexidine, such as Hibisol (ICI). The systematic rubbing of all parts of the hands should continue until all the alcoholic solution has evaporated and the hands are quite dry. This use of a 'surgeon's hand rub' is a satisfactory method of disinfection without the prior use of soap and water, if the hands are not visually soiled.

Protective clothing

Staff who are changing burn dressings should wear a disposable apron and gloves but caps and masks are of little, if any, value in the reduction of cross-infection. Overshoes should not be used; they can easily do more harm than good by becoming a reservoir of bacteria from which the hands are contaminated when changing the overshoes.

The bed-clothes

In addition to frequent changes of linen, it is highly desirable to change the patient's blankets as often as possible, since they rapidly become a reservoir of pathogenic bacteria; efforts should be made to obtain sterilizable cotton blankets, which should be changed at least once a week.

Nose and throat swabs

There is little evidence that staff who are nasal carriers of staphylococci represent any risk to the patients, and it is doubtful whether even streptococcal carriers should be excluded from burn patient care if they are symptom free. It is prudent, however, to ensure that staff with sore throats or skin sepsis are not assigned to patients with burns. It is quite proper to take a throat swab from a staff member with a sore throat since the findings will help in deciding the appropriate treatment for that person. However, it is quite improper to embark upon routine bacteriological monitoring of the staff 'just in case'. Only if there is reasonable clinical suspicion of cross-infection from a staff carrier should that person be asked if he will agree to a swab being taken.

The patient's morale

It is of the utmost importance that all patients should be reassured that their injury is recoverable, even if this is extremely doubtful, and it must be explained to them that there is a time limit to their suffering, and that treatment will follow a well-thought-out and logical plan. Even children of four and five years understand well enough to have this explained to them. Patients often have their favourite nurse, in whom they have most confidence and it is essential that this nurse should understand what is going to happen, roughly when and why. The doctor in charge of the patient should do his utmost to establish a satisfactory mental atmosphere, and a minute or two spent each day in conversation and encouragement will be time well spent. It is quite wrong to minimize the discomforts and the length of time recovery will take, although of course the reverse is also true. When a patient is told firmly that he must expect to be in hospital at least two months, should his burn be extensive and deep, he will quickly accept the position and remain mentally more stable than if he is daily expecting some miraculous cure. Patients should also be reassured that disfigurement and disability will be minimal, although in serious burns of the face and hands some reference should be made to subsequent plastic surgery, which is widely thought by patients to remove scars completely. When the patient has recovered, having undergone a skin grafting session, he will be prepared for the imperfections of plastic surgery if he has had proper advice from the start. During the most trying time of his illness, when skin cover has not yet started or, owing to the extent, is less than half completed, the patient's morale may reach a low ebb and endless encouragement is vital.

It is important to realize that a patient with severe burns will show many of the grief reactions that are commonly associated with bereavement. Indeed, he is actually grieving for his own loss and if the symptoms of this grief are not appreciated, his behaviour may seem bizarre and childish. At first, he may be overwhelmed by the combination of his injury, the strange surroundings and the intensive attention that he is receiving. At this stage he may be quiet and compliant, even withdrawn, but as the intensity of treatment declines at the end of the shock phase, he may become noisy and demanding; frequent requests for seemingly trivial acts – opening or closing the window, adjusting the bed-clothes or the dressings etc. – serve to reassure him that help is still to hand (like the child who, by calling for a drink of water soon after going to bed, is able to reassure himself that someone is there).

The next stage, self-pity, may last for days or weeks. 'Why should this have happened to me?' may be repeated endlessly. There is no satisfactory answer to the question, but sympathetic listening as the patient goes over and over his story is important if he is to move on to the next stage characterized by anger. Whilst the anger will often be directed against those whom he thinks are responsible for his injury, relatives and staff will also become targets. Successful management of this stage requires all staff to recognize the need for this emotional release and help the patient to turn it into a positive drive to get better. The will to survive is vital. The contrary, often seen in the patient who has set fire to himself and does not wish to survive, drags the patient down in spite of the utmost efforts by the staff.

An appreciation of the fact that apparently childish, exceptionally demanding, obstinate or unreasonable behaviour is actually normal following severe burns will go a long way to ensuring that the staff understand and provide the needs of the patient rather than just complaining that he is a 'difficult' patient.

Isolation of the patient adds significantly to his morale problems and to the work of the nursing staff. Nonetheless, isolation may be appropriate if an extensive burn is being treated by exposure, if the patient is very ill or requiring special treatment such as mechanical ventilation, or if there is a high risk of infection to him or other patients. The avoidance of cross-infection between several patients with extensive burns is the rationale for single patient isolation in specialized burns units, but for an individual patient in an ordinary hospital whose burns are being treated with effective antibacterial dressings, isolation is not usually necessary.

Metabolic changes

The abnormal metabolism of patients with extensive burns has been recognized for many years and was well described by Moore and Ball (1952). The negative nitrogen balance that follows all trauma is seen in its severest form in the extensively burned patient and can result in severe weight loss (due mainly to loss of muscle mass) with increased debility, liability to pressure sores, anaemia, hypoproteinuria and greatly enhanced risk of death from sepsis. Untreated, this gross catabolism produces an environment in which all healing processes are seriously retarded; spontaneous epithelialization may cease, skin grafts fail to take, immune mechanisms are suspended and the patient is highly vulnerable to invasive sepsis uncontrollable by antibiotic therapy. Recognition of the importance of minimizing this hypercatabolic tendency is one of the most important advances in the treatment of burns in recent years. It is certain that many patients who succumbed to sepsis in the past did so, not because the appropriate antibiotics were unavailable, but rather because they were in a state of severe metabolic decline in which invasive sepsis was a preterminal event.

Following burn injury, the patient's metabolic rate is greatly increased, the extent of the increase being roughly proportional to the extent and severity of the burn. The generally held view is that the main drive to this hypermetabolism is provided by an abnormally high production of catecholamines (Wilmore, 1974). Although it has not been possible to provide a blockade of this mechanism by drug therapy, Arturson (1978) has shown that by preventing or minimizing a variety of 'stress factors' that may affect the patient, it is possible to reduce the hypermetabolism. These stress factors include noise, discomfort, pain, fear, excitement, heat loss and further trauma.

It is essential, therefore, to minimize pain, discomfort and emotional stress and to provide a quiet and restful environment. Heat loss should be prevented by the provision of a warm environment (30–32 °C), care should be taken to avoid 'cold-stress' during dressing changes and operations and all forms of additional physical trauma should be minimized. Even when all these stresses have been eliminated or minimized, a residual hypermetabolism remains that demands the production of energy from whatever source is available. In the absence of an adequate exogenous source, the available endogenous sources will be utilized. The available carbohydrate reserve is very small and will quickly be consumed to produce energy. Fat stores can then be utilized, but this process of oxidation requires the presence of carbohydrate which will be obtained from the metabolism of muscle protein. If adequate exogenous energy sources are provided, this residual catabolic process can be greatly reduced or even eliminated and the otherwise considerable negative nitrogen balance can be prevented.

Calorie and protein requirements

The total daily intake of calories and protein likely to be needed to prevent significant catabolism and consequential loss of lean body tissue is related to the size of the patient and the size of the burn. Sutherland (1985) has shown that the following schedule is a satisfactory guide for adults.

Calories: 20 per kg body weight + 70 per percentage burn
Protein: 1 g per kg body weight + 3 g per percentage burn.

Thus, a 70-kg patient with 40 per cent of his body surface burned requires 4200 calories and 190 g protein which is at least *double* his requirements if lying in bed uninjured. The optimal ratio of calories to nitrogen is about 130:1 and usually one-half of the non-protein calories are given as carbohydrate and the other half as fat.

Whilst it used to be recommended that burned children would also require greatly increased calorie and protein intakes, more recent work suggests that the intake appropriate for the same age group of healthy children is adequate in the majority of those with burn injury (Sutherland, 1985). A reasonable starting point would be:

Calories: 40 per kg body weight
Protein: 2 g per kg body weight.

These formulae should be looked upon as only giving an indication of the calorie and protein requirement. The actual requirement will vary depending upon the degree to which stress has been reduced or eliminated, the extent of protein loss from the burn wound and the presence or absence of sepsis. The simplest way of monitoring the effectiveness of nutritional support is frequent measurement of the patient's weight. Within 48 hours of burning there will be a marked increase upon the admission weight due to retention of the fluid therapy given during the shock phase. During the next few days there will be a return to admission weight as this fluid is excreted. If no attempt is made to reduce the hypermetabolism, the catabolic process will lead to weight loss of 15–20 per cent of admission weight (in extreme cases even greater loss can occur with death supervening if 25–30 per cent is lost). With proper control of stress and an adequate calorie and protein intake, the weight loss should never exceed 10 per cent and will often be less than 5 per cent. However, over-nutrition is not without risk. Excess carbohydrate intake will be converted to fat and at least in children can lead to fatty degeneration of the liver. Furthermore, the conversion of carbohydrate to fat increases the load of CO_2 that has to be excreted which, in the presence of impaired pulmonary function, could be a serious disadvantage. Excessive protein intake will result in a large nitrogenous load for excretion in the urine and, if renal function is impaired, will enhance the risk of uraemia.

High protein–high calorie enteral feeds

When the protein and calorie requirement of a patient has been calculated, the aim should be to provide it by the enteral route if at all possible. Intravenous or parenteral feeding is necessary occasionally, but is inadvisable as a routine since it enhances the risk of septicaemia in a patient already highly susceptible to this serious complication.

Patients with relatively small burns may be able to take their dietary requirement in the form of 'normal' food and every attempt should be made to provide a palatable and attractive diet with a known nutritional and electrolyte content. The enthusiastic involvement of a dietitian is highly recommended and, if necessary, pressure must be brought to bear upon the hospital management to convince them that the dietary requirement of a burn patient is not a 'hotel service'. Rather it is a vital part of the treatment regimen that can literally determine whether the patient lives or dies. With increasing size of burn, the help of a dietition becomes even more valuable as the provision of supplementary feeds becomes increasingly important. In practice, the patient with extensive burns can seldom eat more than half of his 'normal' intake. Hence, the supplementary feed, perhaps providing three-quarters of the enhanced protein and calorie requirement, becomes the principal method of nutrition and the 'normal' food takes on the supplementary role. However, the provision of good quality food, especially of items that the patient particularly likes, boosts his morale and should not be accorded a low priority simply because it is making a relatively small contribution to the total protein and calorie intake.

In the Yorkshire Regional Burns Centre, a dietitian supervises the dietary requirement of each patient. An appropriate quantity of supplementary feed is manufactured for each patient each day and kept under refrigeration. Portions are removed as required and given to the patient to be drunk from a glass or administered via a nasogastric tube. As shown in *Figures 4.1* and *4.2*, this administration may be either as a bolus at hourly intervals or as a continuous drip using a specially designed pump. The feed is manufactured by adding glucose polymer, fat emulsion and milk protein to fresh pasteurized full-cream milk. The electrolyte content is adjusted as required by the addition of sodium and/or potassium chloride. Milk-shake flavouring may be added immediately prior to

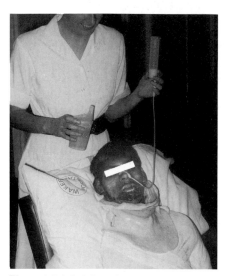

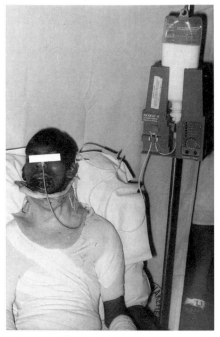

Figure 4.1 Administration of supplementary feed by hourly 'bolus' via nasogastric tube

Figure 4.2 Alternatively, a continuous supply of feed can be given; this is regulated by an electric pump

serving if the feed is to be drunk. Examples of suitable commercial products and the equipment required are shown in *Figure 4.3*.

The production of feeds in-house can be highly cost-effective compared with the use of ready made commercial feeds when it forms part of the routine of a burn centre. The main advantage, however, is the flexibility of the system in providing feeds tailor-made to the particular requirements of the patient; the composition, consistency, concentration and flavour can all be modified as required and problems such as nausea and diarrhoea commonly associated with supplementary feeding can often be prevented or overcome. It is obvious that the production of feeds in bulk necessitates strict attention to hygiene, quality control and storage conditions in order to avoid the possibility of bacterial contamination of the feeds. A great variety of commercial feeds is now available, many of which are suitable for providing the nutritional requirement of the burn patient. These products (examples of which are shown in *Figure 4.4*) fall into three main groups:

(*a*) 'Complete' feeds such as those in cans and bottles in *Figure 4.4* which provide a balanced intake that can, if necessary, replace normal feeding.
(*b*) Supplements such as Build-up (Carnation) that are used to enhance the calorie and protein content of a diet.
(*c*) Additives such as Fortimel (Cow and Gate), Maxisorb and Maxijul (Scientific Hospital Supplies) that increase the intake of one component of the diet. For example, Maxijul added to the patient's drinking water is an easily tolerated way of increasing the daily carbohydrate calorie intake by up to 500 calories in

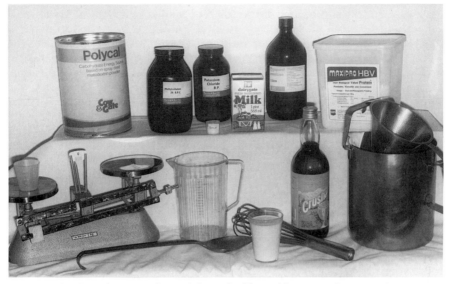

Figure 4.3 Simple equipment and materials required for making up supplementary feed 'in-house'

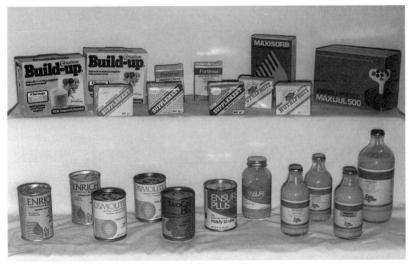

Figure 4.4 The wide variety of commercial preparations available for the treatment of burns

an adult. Commercially prepared feeds are probably the best way of providing the high protein and calorie requirement of the burn patient if a good dietetic service is unavailable of if proper storage of the bulk feed cannot be absolutely guaranteed.

Whatever the source of the supplementary feed, its introduction to the patient must be gradual. Our usual routine is to let the patient drink milk as early as possible, usually by 36 hours after injury. Quarter-strength feed is substituted for the milk next day and the concentration gradually increased until the patient is taking the feed at full concentration – usually by the sixth day after the burn.

If nausea or regurgitation occurs, the volume of feed is temporarily reduced. If diarrhoea occurs, the stool bulk is increased by the addition of methylcellulose to the feed. Should this fail to control the diarrhoea, the next step is to reduce the concentration of the feed. When commercial feeds are being used, a change to another product – for example one with added fibre – may control the intestinal upset. If, in spite of these changes, diarrhoea is troublesome, the use of codeine phosphate or diphenoxylate hydrochloride for a few days is indicated.

The most important factor in minimizing the untoward sequelae of supplementary enteral feeding is the absolute conviction of all concerned that this regimen is an essential part of the treatment. The combination of a cooperative patient, committed nursing staff and an experienced and helpful dietitian will result in a relatively trouble-free nutritional regimen in most cases. The cooperation of the patient is of the utmost value and, in our experience, most adults and many children will drink their feed from a glass when encouraged and supported by nursing staff who are convinced of the importance of adequate nutrition.

Parenteral feeding

Provision of the patient's protein and calorie requirement totally by the intravenous route requires the use of a central venous catheter. However, invasive sepsis is an important cause of death in burn patients and cannula-related sepsis is a very real hazard (Pruitt *et al.*, 1980) that should be avoided whenever possible. Consequently, parenteral nutrition should be employed only when enteral nutrition is clearly ineffective due to severe intolerance or impossible due to paralytic ileus. If the ileus is a consequence of Gram-negative invasive sepsis, the risk associated with central catheterization is even greater, but may be justifiable if a satisfactory nutritional status is to be maintained while the sepsis is brought under control by an appropriate antibiotic. Occasionally, a combination of carbohydrate by the enteral route and the infusion of amino acid solutions and fat emulsion via a peripheral vein may be indicated for a few days when adequate enteral nutrition is proving to be unobtainable.

Transfusions

Late anaemia is common in burns and is thought by some to be more severe if there has been no blood transfusion as part of the treatment of initial shock. In patients with extensive burns, frequent transfusions are usually necessary until skin cover is largely complete. The aim should be to keep the haemoglobin above 12 g/dl. Difficulties are often encountered owing to shortage of suitable veins, but usually cutting down on veins is unnecessary and is to be avoided if possible. It is often easier to erect a transfusion when the patient is anaesthetized, as the veins are more prominent under light anaesthesia, and at this stage transfusions are best combined with the grafting operations. However, if the haemoglobin level has been allowed to fall to 10 g/dl or less, blood transfusion should be undertaken a day or two prior to any surgery or anaesthesia. Lack of suitable veins should not be accepted as an excuse for lack of transfusions. At least two units of blood are usually required to make a significant difference to the haemoglobin level in an adult.

Iron and vitamins

Iron and vitamin therapy should be routine from the end of the shock phase until healing is complete and, possibly, also during the first few weeks after leaving hospital.

Abnormalities of vitamin metabolism occur in burns, and the greater the burn the more is the metabolism of ascorbic acid, thiamin, riboflavin and nicotinamide upset, as evidenced by low plasma concentration and low urinary excretion (Lund et al., 1947). These changes are greatest in the early period, but continue far into the later stages. No evidence has been adduced of increased loss of these vitamins from the burn, and it is presumed that there is in fact a greater requirement than normal; it is known that thiamin, riboflavin and nicotinamide are essential to the enzyme systems that control carbohydrate metabolism, riboflavin is important in amino acid metabolism, and ascorbic acid is necessary for the formation of adrenal cortical hormones.

Similarly, in large burns, there is an increased utilization of iron for erythropoiesis. (There is no advantage to be gained by giving iron injections to burn patients and the enteral route should always be used unless total parenteral feeding is being undertaken.)

For these reasons, vitamin and iron supplements are necessary in patients with large burns, and the following schedule is practicable:

Adults:	Irofol C (Abbott)	1 tablet daily
	Concavit (Wallace Mfg.)	2 capsules daily

If the patient is unable to swallow tablets or is being tube fed, the vitamin and iron supplements need to be given in a soluble form via the nasogastric tube.

Sytron syrup (Parke-Davis)	20 ml daily
Concavit syrup (Wallace Mfg.)	5 ml daily
Vitamin C	500 mg daily
Lexpec (Folic acid syrup: RP Drugs)	1 ml daily

Children: For most children one-half the adult dose will be satisfactory but smaller doses may be appropriate for infants and neonates.

Analgesics, sedatives and hypnotics

The requirement for analgesia during the shock phase of burns is often surprisingly small. With full thickness skin burns there is seldom any complaint of pain because the sensory organs in the skin have also been destroyed. Even when the burns are partial thickness and the survival of sensory end organs can clearly be demonstrated by pinprick, it is unusual for the patient to complain of continuing pain.

However, some patients will complain of pain and most will be affected by fear and discomfort and the provision of analgesia at an early stage is an important part of the treatment. It is common practice in the United Kingdom to administer a narcotic analgesic, such as morphine, while the patient is in the accident department prior to admission or transfer to another hospital. If, in these circumstances, a narcotic appears to be indicated, it *must* be given intravenously, well diluted and in a dose just sufficient to provide immediately the effect required. The dose of morphine would be between 0.1 and 0.2 mg/kg body weight. For this, 10 mg of morphine sulphate should be diluted with water for injection to make a final volume of 10 ml. The syringe *must* be carefully labelled: '*morphine 1 mg/ml*' and it remains the personal responsibility of the doctor until used up or destroyed. An appropriate amount of this morphine solution is slowly injected intravenously until the desired result is achieved.

Morphine, or any other narcotic, should *never* be given subcutaneously to the recently burned patient. It will remain unabsorbed until the circulation improves (possibly several hours later) and may then produce sudden and unexpected depression of breathing and loss of consciousness requiring the urgent administration of naloxone to reverse the narcotic effect. Even intramuscular injections of narcotics may cause similar problems.

During the shock phase, further narcotic analgesia is seldom required and satisfactory sedation, together with anti-emesis, can be provided by *small* doses of chlorpromazine given intravenously and well diluted by the same technique as described above for morphine.

Analgesia for change of dressings can usually be provided most effectively by the patient self-administering Entonox (50 per cent nitrous oxide; 50 per cent oxygen). Quite young children will quickly learn and accept this procedure, particularly if a mouthpiece is used rather than a mask. The gases, premixed in a cylinder, are delivered via a demand valve that opens only when a negative pressure is created on the patient side of the valve, i.e. for gas to flow the patient must be breathing in and the circuit must be airtight. Hence analgesia is provided exactly when it is required, but should the patient become dizzy or start to lose consciousness, the mouthpiece or mask will cease to have an airtight fit and the patient will breathe room air. If the patient is obviously nervous or apprehensive about the impending dressing procedure, 'premedication' with diazepam for adults and trimeprazine for children can be very effective.

In the later stages of management, strong narcotic analgesics are seldom required except in the immediate postoperative period. Indeed, it would be most unwise to give such drugs frequently to a patient who may require treatment for many weeks; addiction consequent upon the frequent prescription of strong narcotic drugs to burned patients has been reported in the USA.

Simple analgesics, such as aspirin and paracetamol, should not be scorned simply because the patient has a big injury. They may well relieve the discomfort of a burn wound or donor site that otherwise could keep the patient restless and promote insomnia. For more severe pain, dihydrocodeine, pentazocine and buprenorphine can be considered. Their effectiveness may vary markedly from patient to patient and some trial and error may be required to establish the most useful drug for a particular patient.

It is important to remember that the maximum cooperation of the patient is required during the day in order that nutritional regimens and physiotherapy procedures can proceed optimally. It is bad practice, therefore, to sedate a patient so that he cannot participate fully in these programmes. Conversely, every attempt should be made to provide a good night's sleep on as many nights as possible. It is all too easy for an 'out-of-phase' cycle to develop in which the patient is restless and demanding at night but then wants to sleep or doze all day. The timing and dosage of sedatives and hypnotics must be adjusted to avoid this unsatisfactory state. Suitable sedative/hypnotics for adults include nitrazepam, diazepam and chlormethiazole with promethazine and trimeprazine being more appropriate for children. Chloral hydrate and chloral derivatives should not be overlooked as relatively safe and useful hypnotics in all age groups.

Antibiotics

A rational and firmly enforced antibiotic policy is essential, both for the management of the individual patient and also to prevent the development of antibiotic-resistant strains of organisms in the environment of the ward. The following policy is that currently followed (1986) in the Yorkshire Regional Burn Centre.

Prophylaxis
The arbitrary and indiscriminate use of antibiotics is counterproductive. Such usage *does not* reduce the risk of serious sepsis; on the contrary it produces selection pressures that promote colonization of both the patient and the environment with resistant organisms or leads to 'superinfection' with yeasts or fungi. However, the prophylactic use of systemic antibiotics is thought to be justified in two specific circumstances.

Streptococcus pyogenes   Early infection of the burn wound with *Strep. pyogenes* is a disaster and prior to the introduction of penicillin used to be life-threatening. Wound infection by this organism can be prevented by a short course (3–5 days) of erythromycin or a β-lactamase stable penicillin, e.g. cloxacillin. (During the last 20 years, all 1600 patients admitted to the Yorkshire Regional Burns Centre have been given this narrow spectrum prophylaxis. Occasionally, *Strep. pyogenes* has been grown from the admission wound swabs but in each case the organism has been absent from subsequent swabs and no clinical evidence of streptococcal infection has been found in these patients.)
    As the general incidence of *Strep. pyogenes* has gradually declined, this prophylactic practice has been abandoned in many burn units. Recently a 'toxic shock syndrome' has been reported as causing mortality and serious morbidity in a few children with small scalds (Frame *et al.*, 1985). A particular strain of *Staph. aureus* – sensitive to erythromycin and cloxacillin – has been implicated and the unit in which this problem occurred has introduced an appropriate prophylaxis policy. There still seems to be merit, therefore, in giving a short course of erythromycin or cloxacillin to all burned patients admitted to hospital and particularly young children with scalds.

'Prophylaxis against invasion'   When surgery has to be carried out on a heavily infected burn wound, bacteraemia occurs that may proceed to septicaemia (Sasaki *et al.*, 1979). Consequently, in these circumstances, and if the wound extends over 30 per cent or more of the body, it is our practice to cover this period by the parenteral administration of an antibiotic selected on the basis of known wound flora. The antibiotics are given with the premedication drugs and continued for three days.

Avoidance of antibiotics
With a few exceptions, e.g. *Strep. pyogenes*, the presence of an organism as a colonist of the burn wound is *not* an indication to give a systemic antibiotic. Indeed, although all our patients have wounds that become colonized by bacteria at some stage, only a small minority receive any antibiotic after the initial prophylaxis described above. For example, 30 per cent of our patients develop *Ps. aeruginosa* infection of their wounds but, in recent years, only 5 per cent of patients have been

given anti-pseudomonas antibiotics (aminoglycosides). It also must be stressed that a moderate pyrexia (38–39 °C) is not by itself an indication to start an antibiotic. The hypermetabolic burn patient, with impaired heat regulating mechanisms, commonly runs a temperature of this order without any signs of invasive sepsis.

Invasive sepsis

Invasive sepsis occurs when pathogenic organisms in the burn wound multiply sufficiently to overcome the body's natural defence mechanisms and then actively invade the living tissues adjacent to the wound. If this advance remains unchecked, septicaemia – active growth of organisms in the blood – is a highly probable sequel. The risk factors in burn wound infection have been reviewed by Pruitt (1984). Patient factors include the extent and depth of the burn, the age of the patient, pre-existing disease and the physical environment of the wound itself. An increased risk is associated with: burn of over 30 per cent body surface area, full thickness skin destruction, infancy and old age, diabetes, cardiopulmonary disease, inhalational injury, obesity and malnutrition, a poor blood supply to the wound and a moist warm wound environment. Microbial factors also influence the balance between resistance and susceptibility to infection. Gram-positive organisms usually predominate in the early days of wound colonization and these are usually confined to the skin and subcutaneous tissues. By the second week, the predominant flora is usually Gram-negative and these organisms are able to proliferate in necrotic tissue and, by entering blood vessels, spread to remote tissues and organs. Invasiveness and virulence are related to the organisms' ability to produce endotoxin, exotoxin, permeability factor and enzymes and to its intrinsic characteristics such as capsule composition and slime production.

An assessment of the general risk of invasive sepsis can be made from consideration of the patient factors detailed above, but awareness of the immediate risk requires knowledge of the appearance of the burn wound, the nature of each type of organism present (genus, strain, substrain and antibiotic sensitivity/ resistance pattern) and, if possible, a measure of the number of organisms present. If the general risk factor is high, it is necessary to inspect the wound on alternate days (or even daily) and keep a detailed record of the microbiology of the wound. Biopsy of the wound has been shown to provide a fairly accurate and reliable assessment of its microbial status. Histological examination and quantitative culture are carried out and a report of 10^5 organisms per gram of tissue is consistent with, although not diagnostic of, invasive burn wound infection (Lindberg, Moncrief and Mason, 1968). In the absence of this specialized technique, reliance must be placed upon conventional wound swabs. After the dressings and all traces of topical antimicrobial agent have been removed, sterile moisturized swabs should be used to sample the wound surface, care being taken to label them accurately, e.g. 'front of left thigh'. The microbiological flora of burn wounds that have been exposed is more difficult to assess; surface swabs may yield no bacterial growth whilst lakes of pus exist beneath the hard dry eschar.

Septicaemia

The diagnosis of septicaemia is essentially clinical taking into account the appearance of the wound, the general demeanour of the patient including anorexia, reluctance to drink, mild confusion or disorientation, and altered trends in the patient's temperature, white cell count and glucose metabolism. Doctors and nurses experienced in burn patient care can often recognize subtle changes in the patient's general condition that are prodromal signs of invasive sepsis. Blood cultures taken at this stage rarely grow any organisms, but the immediate use of an appropriate antibiotic is often proved in retrospect to be justified by the obvious improvement in the patient's condition. If antibiotics are withheld, the prodromal stage of Gram-negative septicaemia may be followed by the sudden onset of septic shock with profound hypothermia, hypotension and multiple organ failure. Recovery is still possible if an effective antibiotic is administered but, if treatment is further delayed, or is ineffective, death will almost certainly supervene.

Choice of antibiotic

Invasive sepsis and septicaemia are rare during the first week post-burn but if they do occur they are much more likely to result from Gram-positive organisms such as *Strep. pyogenes* or *Staph. aureus* than from Gram-negative organisms such as *Ps. aeruginosa*. After the first week the converse is true. However, sepsis may originate from sites other than the burn wound and the possibility of chest infection or urinary tract infection should be considered and appropriately investigated. If antibacterial therapy is required for these infections, broad-spectrum antibiotics are best avoided because of their undesirable effects upon wound flora. Chest infections should be treated with erythromycin or trimethoprim whereas a urinary antiseptic such as nalidixic acid or nitrofurantoin will often be adequate for the treatment of a urinary tract infection.

An infected drip site should not be overlooked as a possible source of organisms responsible for septicaemia. A suspect i.v. cannula or catheter should be carefully removed and sent to the laboratory for culture. Before the results of the culture are known, it should be presumed that the line has been contaminated with wound bacteria and the choice of antibiotic based upon the clinical picture together with knowledge of the wound organisms. Even in the face of obvious septicaemia, blood cultures are positive in less than 10 per cent of such episodes in patients with burns; consequently, blood cultures are of little value in these circumstances.

When the evidence points to the wounds as the probable source of invasive sepsis and the clinical picture is strongly suggestive of a Gram-negative organism being responsible, an aminoglycoside is the antibiotic of choice. If the picture is typical of Gram-positive septicaemia with high core and shell temperatures, delirium and marked leucocytosis, then treatment with cloxacillin, flucloxacillin or fusidic acid would be appropriate. If the origin of the infection is obscure, or the clinician is unable to judge, from the clinical picture, the nature of the organism responsible, a combination of an aminoglycoside (gentamicin, tobramycin, netilmicin, amikacin) plus a carboxypenicillin (ticarcillin) or ureidopenicillin (azlocillin, pipracillin) is likely to be the best first choice. Which particular antibiotics to use should be decided in the knowledge of the resistance patterns of the burn wound flora.

Aminoglycoside antibiotics

In spite of the undoubted activity against *Ps. aeruginosa* of 'third generation' cephalosporins, such as ceftazidime, there is as yet insufficient experience of their use in burn patients to warrant the displacement of aminoglycosides as the main antibiotics for the treatment of Gram-negative septicaemia. Unless the wound swab sensitivity reports suggest otherwise, gentamicin, should be used. (Tobramycin has an activity pattern slightly different from gentamicin and is claimed to be less toxic. Netilmicin is also claimed to be less toxic than gentamicin and is active against some gentamicin-resistant Gram-negative bacilli. Amikacin should be reserved for occasions when a gentamicin-resistant Gram-negative bacillus is thought to be the cause of the septicaemia.) All the aminoglycoside antibiotics mentioned above are both ototoxic and nephrotoxic. They also interfere with neuromuscular blockade. Clearly, great care must be taken to avoid these serious side-effects when aminoglycosides are used. Excretion is principally by way of the kidney and, if there is renal impairment, accumulation occurs in the blood with increased risk of side-effects which are dose related. Consequently, the patient's renal status should be known when these drugs are being used and plasma levels must be measured.

In the absence of significant renal impairment, gentamicin is given by intramuscular or slow intravenous injection at 8-hourly intervals. Plasma concentrations are measured one hour after an intramuscular injection or 20 minutes after an intravenous injection, and also just before the next dose. Peak levels of gentamicin should not exceed 10 µg/ml while the pre-dose (trough) concentrations should be less than 2 µg/ml. If both peak and trough concentrations are low, the dose should be increased; if both are too high, the dose should be decreased. If the peak level is satisfactory but the trough level too high, the dose is correct but the interval between doses should be increased and renal function carefully examined. When renal function is impaired, the interval between doses is increased according to the following schedule: creatinine clearance 30–70 ml/min, dose interval 12 hours; 10–30 ml/min, 24 hours; 5–10 ml/min, 48 hours, less than 5 ml/min, after each dialysis or at 3–4 day intervals.

Experience of using gentamicin for long periods (several weeks) has shown that impairment of renal function gradually occurs in spite of satisfactory peak and trough levels. An early warning of this tubular damage is afforded by quantitative urinalysis that measures small protein molecules and enzymes not normally present in the urine (Yu et al., 1983).

The normal dose of gentamicin is 2–5 mg/kg daily in divided doses every 8 hours. However, the altered antibiotic pharmacokinetics in burn patients can easily lead to subtherapeutic treatment (Zaske, Sawchuk and Gerding, 1976) and plasma levels should be monitored at 2-day intervals. To obviate suboptimal levels in the early stages of treatment, Harburchak and Pruitt (1978) have recommended a loading dose of twice the normal dose and subsequent maintenance doses 1.5 times the normal until plasma concentrations are measured on the second day of therapy.

Specific local infections

Three types of infection occurring the later stages deserve mention.

Firstly, late streptococcal infection can supervene even when the burn is almost healed, and unexplained redness or swelling of a limb should be treated energetically on the assumption that this is a dangerous streptococcal manifestation until proved otherwise. Secondly, *Bacillus proteus* infection of the wound may, especially in combination with a staphylococcus, result in very delayed epithelialization, with complete loss of skin grafts in an area which looks reasonably clean. If careful inspection reveals slight undermining of the edges of discrete raw areas, proteus infection should be suspected, and local applications of polymyxin or chlorhexidine will usually clear the infection within a few days. Proteus infection is likely to remain local and represents a nuisance rather than a danger to life. Thirdly, in very rare cases, an area that has proved to be completely unreceptive to skin grafts, and is not infected by *Pseudomonas pyocyaneus, Proteus* or *Streptococcus* sp., may be found to grow *Candida albicans* in culture, in which case dressings impregnated with nystatin will rapidly improve the position.

Steroids

At the present time, no convincing evidence has been put forward that burns patients benefit from the administration of corticosteroids in the early stages of their illness and we believe that they are to be avoided. The administration of anabolic steroids in the later stages of the illness has been advocated, but their usefulness has not been proven and they may indeed be dangerous in patients with large infected wounds. At a later stage, usually after five or six weeks, if stubborn unhealed areas still remain, especially with oedematous granulation, or when the grafted areas look as though secondary breakdown is occurring, local steroid applications (e.g. hydrocortisone either alone or in conjunction with neomycin or tetracycline) are sometimes successful.

Antitoxins and vaccines

In 1956, Federov and his associates in the USSR reported beneficial results when the serum from patients convalescent from burns was infused to patients acutely ill with recent burns. Although much research effort has been expended in this direction since that time, it is still not certain if these and subsequent results were due to the presence of antibodies against a specific burns toxin, against a general trauma toxin, or against bacterial toxins. The most encouraging studies of vaccines have been carried out by Jones and Roe. They have spent many years developing and perfecting a polyvalent pseudomonas vaccine and, after preliminary trials in the UK, were able to mount a full scale trial in Dehli (Jones, Roe and Gupta, 1980). The vaccine was successful in reducing mortality in the vaccine-treated group to about one-quarter of that in the non-vaccine group. Unfortunately, the vaccine is still not available commercially.

Zinc

It is thought that zinc is necessary for the satisfactory healing of wounds, and zinc deficiency has been reported as a cause of poor or delayed wound healing. If final healing is delayed it may be worth trying zinc supplements. The dose for children under 3 years is zinc sulphate 110 mg in milk three times daily; for older children and adults, zinc sulphate 220 mg in milk three times daily (Larsen *et al.*, 1970).

Prevention of avoidable complications

In common with other patients who are seriously ill for protracted periods, burn patients are particularly liable to the following complications.

Pressure sores

Extensive pressure sores may well tip the balance against recovery. Frequent shifts of position, especially in the elderly, are essential, and the use of low air loss beds, fluidized bead beds or ripple beds should be considered where pressure sores are feared. Active nursing care is of the greatest importance.

Urinary sepsis

In burns involving the buttocks and thighs in females, it is often necessary to resort to the indwelling catheter for some weeks, to minimize soiling of the raw area and to protect recently applied skin grafts. It is essential that sterile technique is scrupulous when the catheter is inserted or changed, and frequent routine culture of the urine is obligatory, so that the appropriate antimicrobial agent can be prescribed if infection supervenes. Pyelonephritis is a common finding at postmortem in burns, and faulty treatment here is very dangerous. There is no doubt that catheters should be avoided if possible, although they are frequently necessary during the shock phase for assessment of the patient's fluid balance; if the catheter can be dispensed with when shock is over, so much the better.

Oral sepsis

Strict attention to oral hygiene is of course important when the burn involves the lips, mouth or air passages. An occasional complication of any large burn, however, especially if considerable quantities of antibiotics have been given, is extensive thrush of the mouth, oesophagus and pharynx, and this condition has proved fatal on more than one occasion in young children. The throat should, therefore, be examined daily, and nystatin administered if candidiasis is found.

Diarrhoea

Diarrhoea can be very debilitating and dangerous in a patient already sufficiently ill. While this is not the place for a full discussion of diarrhoeas in general, it can be said that in burns cases the diarrhoea is most often dietetic, due to the aperient effect of the high protein supplements. Modification of the diet, as mentioned earlier in this chapter, should be tried first. If this fails to control the diarrhoea, drugs such as codeine phosphate and diphenoxylate hydrochlorate may be given. Less often, the diarrhoea may be a side-effect of an orally administered antibiotic such as tetracyline and, rarely, may be a consequence of colonization of the colon with *Clostridium difficile* which may develop after antibiotic therapy. The condition is known as pseudomembranous colitis and causes the patient to be very ill. Oral vancomycin or metronidazole are said to be the specific treatment. Finally, bacterial enteritis – the causative organism coming from the wound or, possibly, contaminated feed – should not be overlooked as a possible cause of diarrhoea in burn patients.

Wasting of muscles

General physiotherapy to all limbs which are not of necessity immobilized by the burn, and breathing exercises, both help the patient during the acute illness and shorten the period of debility when recovery is far enough advanced to start getting out of bed. It is particularly important to prevent footdrop, which is very common, especially in burns of the legs.

Summary

By way of summary, consideration should be given to what can be done for a patient whose condition is rapidly deteriorating some three weeks after sustaining an extensive burn.

(1) Is he septicaemic? Look at the 4-hourly temperature chart – a high swinging temperature means staphylococcal septicaemia, a moderate sustained temperature means Gram-negative invasion. Intravenous gentamicin is the drug of choice with the addition of ticarcillin if there is no obvious improvement in 12 hours. Have a look at the burn – are there pockets of pus under the sloughs? If so, evacuate them and get rid of as much slough as possible.
(2) Is there sepsis of the urinary tract or the respiratory tract? If there is treat it.
(3) Is the patient grossly anaemic? Carry out a full blood count and transfuse him.
(4) Does the patient have diarrhoea? If so why? Treat it.
(5) What is the state of his nutrition? Is his intake satisfactory?
(6) Listen to his chest. Is he dying of pulmonary oedema, or because he cannot cough up his secretions? If he is, do a tracheostomy. Suck out the secretions and give him physiotherapy day and night.
(7) Never give up. He is not dying of some mysterious toxin associated with burns but of some definite pathological process which can be diagnosed and may be treatable.

References

ARTURSON, M. G. S. (1978) Metabolic changes following thermal injury. *World Journal of Surgery*, **2,** 203–213

FEDEROV, N. A. (1956) In *Proceedings of the 6th Congress. International Society for Blood Transfusion.* p. 44. Basle: S. Karger

FRAME, J. D., EVE, M. D., HACKETT, M. E. J., DOWSETT, E. G., BRAIN, A. N., GAULT, D. T. et al. (1985) The toxic shock syndrome in burned children. *Burns,* **11,** 234–241

HABURCHAK, D. R. and PRUITT, B. A. Jr (1978) Use of systemic antibiotics in burned patients. *Surgical Clinics of North America,* **58,** 1119–1132

JONES, R. J., ROE, E. A. and GUPTA, J. L. (1980) Controlled trials of pseudomonas immunoglobulin and vaccine in burned patients. *Lancet,* **ii,** 1263–1265

LARSEN, D. L., MAXWELL, R., ABSTON, S. and DOBROKOWSKI, M. (1970) Zinc deficiency in burned children. *Plastic and Reconstructive Surgery,* **40,** 13

LINDBERG, R. B., MONCRIEF, J. A. and MASON, A. D. Jr (1968) Control of experimental and clinical burn wound sepsis by topical application of sulfamylon compounds. *Annals of the New York Academy of Science,* **150,** 950

LUND, C. C., LEVENSON, S. M., GREEN, R. W., PAIGE, R. W., ROBINSON, P. E., ADAMS, M. A. et al. (1947) Ascorbic acid, thiamine, riboflavine and nicotinic acid in relation to acute burns in man. *Archives of Surgery,* **55,** 557

MOORE, F. D. and BALL, M. R. (1952) *The Metabolic Response to Surgery*. Springfield, Ill.: C. C. Thomas

PRUITT, B. A. Jr (1984) The diagnosis and treatment of infection in the burn patient. *Burns,* **11,** 79–91

PRUITT, B. A. Jr, McMANUS, W. F., KIM, S. H. and TREAT, R. C. (1980) Diagnosis and treatment of cannula related intravenous sepsis in burn patients. *Annals of Surgery,* **191,** 546–554

SASAKI, T. M., WELCH, G. W., HERNDON, D. N., KAPLAN, J. Z., LINDBERG, R. B. and PRUITT, B. A. Jr (1979) Burn wound manipulation-induced bacteraemia. *Journal of Trauma,* **19,** 46–48

SUTHERLAND, A. B. (1985) Nutrition and general factors influencing infection in burns. *Journal of Hospital Infection,* **6** (Suppl. B), 31–42

TAYLOR, L. J. (1978) Evaluation of hand washing techniques. *Nursing Times,* **74,** 54–55

WILMORE, D. W. (1974) Nutrition and metabolism following thermal injury. In *Clinics in Plastic Surgery*. Ed. J. A. Moncrief, pp. 603–619. Philadelphia: W. B. Saunders

YU, H., COOPER, E. H., SETTLE, J. A. D. and MEADOWS, T. (1983) Urinary protein profiles after burn injury. *Burns,* **9,** 339–349

ZASKE, D. E., SAWCHUK, R. J. and GERDING, D. N. (1976) Increased dosage requirements of gentamicin in burn patients. *Journal of Trauma,* **16,** 824–828

Chapter 5

Burns of special areas

Face, head and neck

In any burn involving the head and neck, special efforts must be made at the initial examination to determine if the air passages or the eyes have been damaged as this may alter the priorities of treatment.

The eyes, mouth and throat can be inspected; hoarseness or respiratory distress indicate damage to the respiratory tract.

In any burn of the face, oedema is marked, and the eyelids often become so swollen that the eyes are completely closed (*Figures 5.1* and *5.2*). They should therefore be examined as soon as possible and before the oedema develops, using an eyelid retractor if necessary. If the lids are already swollen when the patient is

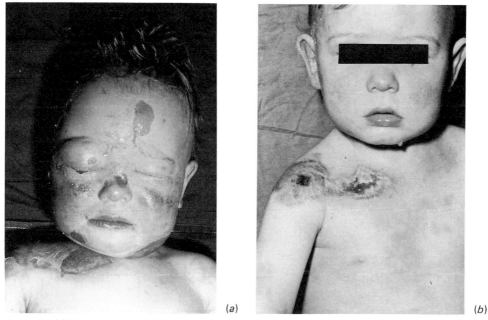

(a)   (b)

Figure 5.1 (*a*) Even a very superficial scald of the face can result in marked oedema. (*b*) Eight days later healing is almost complete.

113

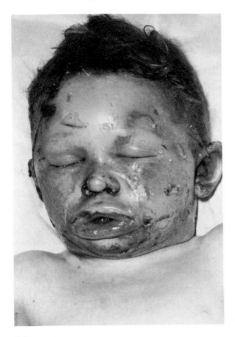

(a)

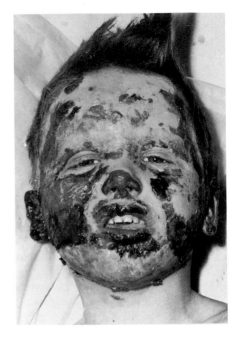

(b)

(c)

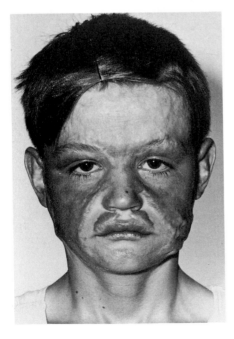

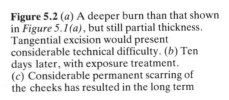

Figure 5.2 (a) A deeper burn than that shown in *Figure 5.1(a)*, but still partial thickness. Tangential excision would present considerable technical difficulty. (b) Ten days later, with exposure treatment. (c) Considerable permanent scarring of the cheeks has resulted in the long term

first seen, the oedema fluid can be temporarily displaced by gentle pressure and massage for long enough to examine the eyes. If the eye is damaged, an ophthalmological opinion must be obtained without delay.

Burns of the face and neck are usually treated by exposure, partly because bandaging of this area adds extra distress to the patient.

Superficial burns
Superficial burns heal well and surface crusting can be expected to loosen after 8–10 days. Loose crusts are gently cleaned off or snipped away as necessary and, provided the area remains dry and free of sepsis, often no mark of the burn will remain after a few more days.

Deep partial thickness burns
Deep partial thickness burns of the face are best treated by tangential excision, in the same way as are other areas of the body. It can sometimes be very difficult to decide if tangential excision of a burn of the face is really required; operation involves considerable blood loss, and is technically more difficult than tangential excision of a large flat surface. Nevertheless under certain circumstances – a fit patient, definite loss of sensation to pinprick confirmed by serial examinations and good operating facilities with adequate available operating time – tangential excision of facial or scalp burns pays handsome dividends in minimizing scarring and disfiguring contractures. Hair follicles can be preserved, lying as they do in the depths of the skin and the upper layers of the subcutaneous tissue (Roberts, 1983).

Full thickness burns
If well demarcated, these are also best treated by primary excision and skin graft, but often this course of action is precluded by the overall extent of the burn or the patient's poor general condition. Early grafting on clean granulating areas is also usually very satisfactory and often to be preferred, but any delay in providing skin cover on a fresh granulating area will be heavily penalized by gross fibrosis and disfiguring contracted scars especially around the lips and eyelids, and on the front of the neck (*see Figures 5.2 and 5.3*).

Eyelids

Although eyelid skin is very thin it often escapes serious damage owing to spasm of the orbicularis oculi at the time of the accident. In peacetime the commonest cause of eyelid burns is an epileptic fit or a fainting attack during which the patient falls unconscious on to a fire (Schofield, 1954).

The importance of eyelid burns lies in the fact that retraction of the lids, with resulting exposure of the cornea, readily develops and this may quickly result in corneal ulceration, perforation and loss of the eye. It is of immense importance to realize that damage to the eye is usually entirely due to this retraction and is not caused primarily by the injury. It should always be possible to prevent this damage to the eye by being constantly alert to the danger and acting without delay as soon as treatment is indicated.

Exposure of the cornea may occur at the following times:

(1) When the first crust has formed and by its rigidity prevents the lids from closing properly.

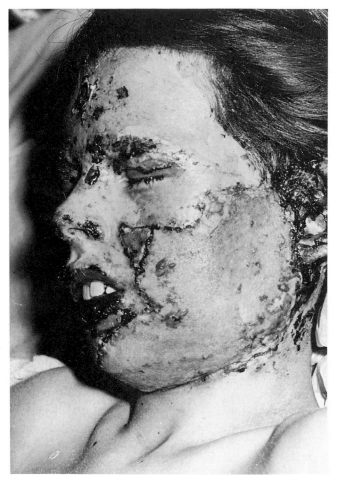

Figure 5.3 Grafting early on granulating areas gives good results. Every effort should be made to resurface wounds of the face with large sheets of skin to avoid junctional scarring

(2) Almost as soon as the granulations are formed, scar contracture commences, and lid retraction may occur in granulating full thickness burns before grafts are applied.
(3) Grafted lids soon contract and further grafting is almost invariably necessary at an early date.

The treatment of eyelid burns is, therefore, usually as follows:

(*a*) Initial treatment is, as for burns of the face in general, by exposure.
   The eyes often discharge copiously and frequent cleansing by wiping with wet swabs is needed.
   When crusts have formed, they are inspected daily to see that lid closure is adequate and the cornea is protected. If inadequate closure is noticed, because of hardness of the crusts, they should be softened by massage with soft paraffin.
(*b*) Partial thickness burns require no further treatment when the crusts have separated.

(*c*) If the burn is of full thickness depth, the slough soon becomes apparent and separates rapidly.

The separation should be encouraged by frequent wet dressings moistened with saline, rather than eusol which tends to sting the eyes.

As soon as the granulations are healthy, split skin grafts are applied. These grafts may be exposed, or covered by dressings and bandaged, whichever seems convenient. No attempt is made at this time to stretch the lids over stent moulds or other materials, for the lid margin is very friable and stitches easily cut through, resulting in unsightly notching.

These first grafts soon contract and further grafting must be performed if the cornea is again in danger. This second grafting usually has to be performed about four weeks after the first. The lid margins are by then firm and hold stitches well.

(*d*) It is best to perform this secondary grafting of upper and lower eyelids at separate sessions in order to achieve maximum correction. Upper eyelids should be operated on first, as they are much more important than the lower lids in covering the cornea.

The lids are incised transversely above the lashes well out beyond the medial and lateral canthi, and dissection continued between skin and muscle until the lid can be markedly overcorrected.

The raw area is then covered by a split-skin graft, and then stretched over a mould of stent composition by tension sutures, so that the maximum amount of skin graft is supplied. This is the classical 'outlay graft' as described by Sir Harold Gillies (1920).

The lower lids are corrected as soon as the upper lid grafts are well established and, if possible, post-auricular Wolfe grafts are used to give the best permanent repair.

(*e*) Tarsorrhaphy:

It will be noticed that in the above description, no mention has been made of tarsorrhaphy. If the programme is carried through satisfactorily, tarsorrhaphy is unnecessary and indeed grafting of the lids is more easily performed in the absence of tarsorrhaphy.

Nevertheless there is no doubt that a tarsorrhaphy will protect the cornea satisfactorily and may be indicated in some cases:

(i) When facilities for continuous skilled supervision and grafting are not available. If this is likely to be the case tarsorrhaphy must be performed within a few days of injury so that it will be firmly established before scar contracture begins. Once healed, a tarsorrhaphy will hold indefinitely, although the scar may stretch and it will be necessary to insert more skin before the lids are separated.

(ii) When part of the full thickness of the upper eyelid has been destroyed a tarsorrhaphy combined with grafting of the skin defect is almost always necessary.

(*f*) Neglected cases – excision and grafting as an emergency measure.

If there has been a delay of some days, and the cornea has become exposed by shrinkage of the coagulated eyelid skin, it may be necessary to excise the dead tissue surgically; this will release the eyelid to provide cover. The raw area is then covered with a skin graft; as stated above further grafting is usually necessary at an early date.

If the full thickness of the eyelid is destroyed, tarsus, conjunctiva and all, then the eye itself may be severely damaged and enucleation may be necessary. This is rare.

It cannot be too strongly emphasized that burns in the region of the eye take priority over all other areas; keratitis due to exposure must *never* be allowed to occur. If the surgeon in charge of the case feels unable to give proper treatment to the eyelids, then help must be obtained, and until such help is available, neomycin and hydrocortisone eyedrops should be instilled 4-hourly, or the eye protected with a bland cream (e.g. lanette wax) to prevent the cornea becoming dry.

Ears

Full thickness burns of the ears are relatively common; the helix is frequently deeply burned in flash accidents and conflagrations, and the whole ear in epileptic attacks. If the whole ear is burnt and is hard to the touch and completely white, it should be excised. If the helix only is burnt, then it is best to await developments. With luck, the burn may not actually expose the cartilage during its sloughing phase, in which case the final deformity of the ear will be minimal. If the cartilage becomes exposed, an extremely painful chondritis with gross oedema and discharge may ensue, and can 'reduce resolute men to weeping wrecks' (McIndoe, 1983). If untreated, the chondritis will result in loss of about half the cartilage of the ear, which then heals as a crumpled appendage. At the first sign of chondritis, the rim of the ear should be opened up and all the exposed cartilage excised, making sure that there is healthy tissue to cover the cut edge; the skin is then loosely approximated and a drain left in. Deformity of the ear will result but will be less extensive than if the condition is left untreated.

Nose

Full thickness skin destruction of the nose is uncommon, except in epileptic burns. If the cartilage is burnt, extensive deformity is inevitable, so that generally conservative treatment is the rule, with grafting of the granulating area when it is ready. It is often necessary in the early stages, however, to pick away the crusts from the nostrils to facilitate nasal breathing. Plastic reconstruction may be indicated later on, though for the elderly patient a prosthesis may be best.

Lips

Burns of the lips usually heal rapidly, although they may cause great distress in the first few days. Oral hygiene is important, and anaesthetic creams such as benzocaine compound ointment BPC may alleviate the pain to some extent.

Burns of the upper airway

Burns of the upper airway, resulting from the inhalation of flame and hot gases, are almost always associated with obvious burning of the skin around the nose and mouth. Hence, when a patient is admitted with burns in the nostrils and/or inside the lips, a close examination and careful assessment of the air passages is essential.

If flame or hot gases have reached the larynx and upper trachea, airway obstruction due to laryngeal oedema is inevitable. This obstruction may be preceded by hoarseness and stridor but sometimes occurs suddenly with very little warning. Even without obvious thermal damage to the laryngeal airway, it is possible for laryngeal oedema to develop secondary to generalized burn oedema of the face, oropharynx and neck. It is essential, therefore, to re-assess, at half-hour (or even quarter-hour) intervals during the early post-burn period, the state of the upper airway in all patients with burns or scalds of the face and neck.

Upper airway obstruction may result from the pressure effect of burn oedema in the neck. Mild obstruction may be cured by extension of the head; a suitable pad placed under the shoulders and base of the neck may suffice. When the burn oedema is associated with full thickness skin burns of the neck, the effect is that of strangulation and dramatic relief of the obstruction follows surgical release of the tension by means of scalpel incisions through the leathery burn eschar.

When careful observation indicates that upper airway obstruction due to laryngeal oedema is likely to develop, endotracheal intubation should be undertaken without delay. It cannot be too strongly emphasized that procrastination will result in the procedure of intubation becoming progressively more difficult, and eventually impossible. Once actual laryngeal obstruction has reached the point of producing asphyxia, an emergency tracheostomy may have to be performed in the next few minutes if the patient's life is to be saved. Should this obstruction occur whilst the patient is undergoing transfer from the accident department to the ward or to another hospital, the outcome is likely to be fatal. Consequently, no burn patient in whom endotracheal intubation is indicated should leave the accident department until the airway is secure.

The intubation should be performed by a skilled and experienced anaesthetist since it is much more difficult in the presence of oedema than when the upper airways are normal. A pre-oxygenation, thiopentone and muscle relaxant technique will be appropriate in many instances, but different techniques (including conscious intubation) may be indicated in other cases. The knowledge and experience required to decide which technique is appropriate in the particular circumstances, and the degree of skill necessary to carry out the intubation itself, should not be underestimated.

Modern endotracheal tubes can safely be left *in situ* for several days. Where upper airway obstruction is the only problem, this period will allow the resolution of the oedema at which time the tube can be removed. Even when damage to the lower airways by smoke inhalation requires treatment by mechanical ventilation, the endotracheal tube will suffice in most cases. However, if ventilation is to be prolonged for more than a few days, or severe burns (particularly of the face) are to be treated by surgical intervention (possibly on several occasions) during the first week, a semipermanent bypass of the orolaryngeal airway may be indicated in which case tracheostomy should be performed. In babies and adults, this can be performed under local anaesthesia if necessary, but in children over one year general anaesthesia is essential. The operation is performed as follows:

(1) Infiltrate the lower part of the neck between the sternomastoid muscles with about 20 ml of xylocaine with adrenaline. If operating entirely with local anaesthesia, use 1.25 per cent xylocaine with 1 in 80 000 adrenaline. If operating under general anaesthesia, use 0.5 per cent xylocaine with 1 in 200 000 adrenaline.

(2) Extend the patient's neck, making sure there is no rotation of the head.
(3) Incise the skin, transversely if time permits, or vertically if speed is essential. The incision should be 2.5 cm long and centred on a point 1.5 cm above the suprasternal notch.
(4) Deepen the incision by blunt dissection between the strap muscles in the midline. The trachea can be easily felt with the tip of the finger.
(5) Clear the soft tissues off the front of the trachea, if necessary retracting the thyroid isthmus or dividing the isthmus between clamps.
(6) Insert a sharp hook into the cricoid and pull upwards to hold the trachea steady.
(7) Incise the trachea. The method of incision differs in children and adults. In adults, cut a rectangular trap-door flap, base downwards, which when hinged back, will leave an aperture sufficiently large to accept the tracheostomy tube. Stitch the trapdoor flap of trachea to the lower margin of the skin wound with a single catgut stitch. In children, do not cut a flap because this can lead to stenosis; instead, make a simple longitudinal incision from the second tracheal ring, downwards.
(8) Retract the edges of the wound in the trachea; ask the anaesthetist to withdraw the endotracheal tube as far as necessary and gently insert the tracheostomy tube; tie the tapes at the back of the neck. Tie the tapes in a knot, not in a bow, to avoid confusion with the tapes of the gown. If the tube is displaced, it may be extremely difficult to re-insert.
(9) If a large skin incision has been made, suture the skin edges where the wound projects beyond the flange of the tracheostomy tube.

Postoperatively, it is essential that the inspired air should be humidified to avoid drying of secretions. The tracheostomy tube should be kept clear by frequent suction, and physiotherapy given. It is a good rule that the tracheostomy tube should be changed for a clean one every 48 hours, and this procedure should be medically supervised, not left to the nursing staff. The tracheostomy tube should be removed when direct or indirect laryngoscopy shows that oedema of the upper respiratory tract has subsided. Antibiotics should be given intensively, as septic bronchopneumonia is almost inevitable and carries a high mortality.

Burns of the scalp

Except in epileptics, the full thickness of the scalp is seldom destroyed. Burns of the scalp are usually treated conservatively by exposure, after clipping short or shaving the hair.

In epileptics who have been burned, however, destruction of the full thickness of the scalp is common. These burns are typically well demarcated and obviously deep, and are suitable for early excision and grafting (*Figure 5.4*). When the scalp has been excised, the pericranium is carefully examined. If it is viable, split-skin grafts should be applied immediately. It is important that the exposed pericranium should not be left unprotected, for it readily dries, and dies (Harrison, 1952).

If the pericranium is dry and brown, then it is dead, and this means that the outer table of the skull will also be non-viable. The surgeon can then follow one of two courses:

(i) He can remove the outer table of the skull with chisel and hammer (Craig), exposing vascular diploë. This layer will soon produce granulations which will

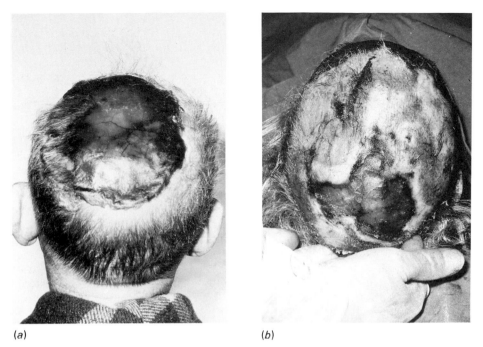

(a)   (b)

Figure 5.4 (*a*) Full thickness burn of the scalp sustained by lying unconscious near the fire for a prolonged period. (*b*) Full thickness burn of the scalp due to being in close proximity to a radiant heat source (Bradford Football Stand Fire, 1985); early excision and skin grafting is indicated

support grafts, although it is difficult to produce a uniform surface with one operation, and further minor sequestrectomies and grafts are often necessary.

(ii) He can leave the outer table of the skull exposed until it has been loosened as a natural sequestrum by the development of a layer of granulations in the vascular diploë. This may take a very long time (up to a year) and such a long period of disability should be avoided if possible, at any rate in younger patients.

The neck

Skin loss on the front of the neck is common and, if extensive, will lead to severe contracture unless special steps are taken. If medium thickness split-skin grafts are placed on the granulations after three weeks or so, marked contraction takes place and cannot be prevented by splintage. Subsequent plastic reconstruction, usually by means of pedicled skin flaps, becomes necessary. Similarly, once a thick layer of granulation tissue forms on and in the platysma muscle, gross shrinkage of the fibrous tissue will occur as it matures.

If other circumstances are favourable, we believe it is well worthwhile to try to avoid this sequence of events by carrying out a definitive repair at an early stage (*Figure 5.5*). The skin of the neck is thin, so that separation of the slough occurs early and it may be possible to place a thick skin graft on minimal granulations as early as the fifteenth day after burning. The graft is taken from the trunk or buttock, often with a Padgett's dermatome, and sutured into place. The operation

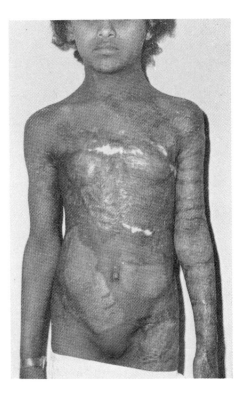

Figure 5.5 Full thickness burn of the neck treated by maximal-thickness dermatome graft applied to the granulating area on the fifteenth day after burning. *No secondary surgery has been required.* Note donor site scar on abdomen. (This photograph was taken 4 years post-burn)

is undertaken as a separate procedure well in advance of the main skin grafting sessions. If such a thick graft is taken, it has to be accepted that the donor site will not be re-usable for many weeks, if at all, and thus if a donor site on the trunk or buttocks is not available, or if it is thought that every scrap of available autograft will be needed on several subsequent occasions, this type of early neck cover cannot be undertaken.

Some surgeons advocate that, after grafting the neck, a moulded splint should be constructed and worn continuously for many months to prevent shrinkage of the skin grafts. We are not convinced that this type of splintage is always necessary, nor that it is invariably effective.

The arms

It is difficult to treat burns of the arms by exposure owing to the problem of avoiding contact with the bedclothes. In the early stages, the limb should be elevated to minimize oedema. If the burn is deep and extends around the whole circumference of the limb, there is the danger of a tourniquet effect developing, leading to embarrassment of the circulation. This is particularly liable to occur with deep, dry, hard burns and, in this type of case, it is essential that the burned skin should be incised longitudinally throughout its full extent to relieve tension. Since the skin is dead, this is easily done without any anaesthesia and the wound will gape widely. An antiseptic dressing is then applied and the arm elevated.

The hands

Burns of the hands have an importance out of proportion to the size of the area involved and often lead to serious disability which can be greatly aggravated by inefficient early treatment.

The principles of treatment are similar to those for burns elsewhere, but special problems arise because:

(i) An extent of scarring which elsewhere would be insignificant, may cause serious disability in the hands.
(ii) Deep structures, such as tendons and joints, are often damaged or endangered in burns of the hand and special methods of repair may be necessary at an early stage if maximum function is to be preserved.

The following points are important in treatment:

(a) Circumferential burns often produce a leathery eschar which may act like a tourniquet and result in ischaemic gangrene of the digits. These burns should therefore be decompressed by longitudinal incisions.
(b) A burned hand readily assumes a position which can lead to serious secondary damage, and this must be avoided by correct splintage (see below).
(c) Burned hands become oedematous and, if the oedema is allowed to persist, it results in fibrosis and limitation of movement. This oedema can be minimized by high elevation. The amount of oedema on the dorsum of the hand and fingers in a burn of doubtful depth is a good indication of the severity of the burn; if there is considerable oedema the deeper dermis is probably damaged and loss of pinprick sensation will confirm the need for early tangential excision (see below). During the early stages, movement increases the oedema, and this is another reason for splintage as part of the initial treatment.
(d) As soon as the hand is healed, active movements must be encouraged. Severe burns, no matter how well treated, result in stiffness and active rehabilitation is always necessary.
(e) Exposure treatment is unsuitable except for obviously superficial burns, and the treatment of choice for all severe hand burns is by dressings.
(f) Deep partial or full thickness destruction of the thin skin of the dorsum of the hand is common. The extensor tendons escape serious damage at the time of injury, but often become oedematous. The hand, if unsplinted, tends to go into a position of full extension at the metacarpophalangeal joints and full flexion at the interphalangeal joints. In this position, the oedematous extensor tendons are stretched tightly over the dorsal aspects of the proximal interphalangeal joints and may undergo ischaemic necrosis, thus exposing the joints. This danger is greatest over the first 4–5 days and it is important that during this period the proximal interphalangeal joints should be held in full extension. The metacarpophalangeal joints are not at risk during this stage, but if they remain in extension for more than 10 days, they easily become stiff in this position and it may be impossible to regain flexion (Braithwaite and Watson, 1949). Failure of treatment at this stage may lead to permanent deformity of the hand (Figure 5.6, which shows a typical 'boutonnière' deformity of the proximal interphalangeal joint due to destruction of the middle slip of the extensor tendon, and fixed extension of the metacarpophalangeal joints). It was previously our opinion that the hand should be splinted from the

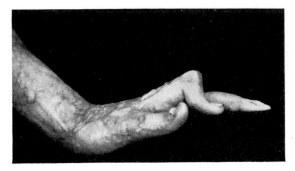

Figure 5.6 Fixed extension of the metacarpophalangeal joints and fixed flexion of proximal interphalangeal joint due to a dorsal burn

commencement of treatment in the ideal position for both sets of joints, i.e. with the proximal interphalangeal joints in flexion. Further experience has convinced us that, in the early stages, it is extremely difficult to maintain this position. Since there is no anxiety about the metacarpophalangeal joints during the first few days, it is easier to protect the vulnerable interphalangeal joints if the hand is initially splinted with the fingers in full extension at all joints. After 4–7 days, when the oedema has subsided and the danger to the proximal interphalangeal joints is past, the metacarpophalangeal joints can be brought down into flexion.

Hands are burned in certain types of accident and the burns therefore tend to follow specific patterns according to the type of injury. The following types can be recognized:

(1) Flash burns.
(2) Flame burns.
(3) Contact burns.
(4) Crush burns.

Flash burns

These are common injuries and usually result from industrial accidents, such as petrol explosions, power station mishaps and blowbacks from furnaces.

The mechanism of the accident is such that the exposure to heat is of very short duration; it may be long enough to destroy the thin skin on the dorsum of the hand, but the thick skin of the palm always escapes destruction. The palmar skin is usually further protected by the normal position of the hand during working, i.e. in pronation with flexion of the fingers.

Treatment
It is often difficult to be certain of the depth of skin damage, and treatment should therefore be conservative for the first two days, which will allow for further clinical assessment. An early decision must, however, be taken regarding the indications for and against tangential excision. As soon as convenient, the hand must be carefully examined in a good light. If there is no oedema, and the patient can fully flex and extend his fingers, the burn is almost certainly very superficial. If there is a degree of oedema, limiting the full excursion of the fingers especially of the

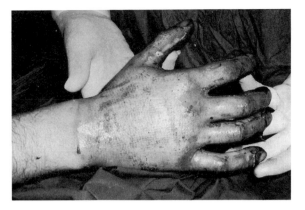

(a)

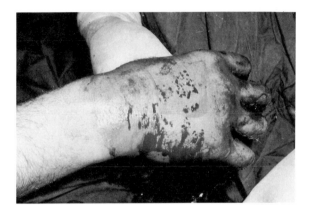

(b)

(c)

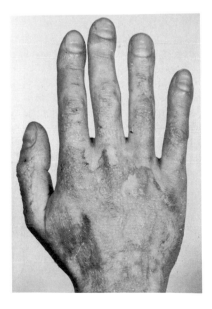

Figure 5.7 (*a*) Flash burn of the back of the hand and fingers. Note some oedema indicating probable deep dermal involvement. Pinprick sensation was absent. (*b*) Tangential excision reveals capillary bleeding at a fairly superficial level. The excision does not need to go any deeper than this. It is important to include excision of damaged skin on the fingers. (*c*) Healed fully mobile hand on the fourteenth day after burning. Note numerous tiny inclusion cysts, which can be treated by pricking or squeezing. The tendency to cyst formation, which is greatest when the burn has been relatively superficial (as here), disappears after several weeks

metacarpophalangeal joints, examination by the pinprick test is essential (*see Figure 5.7*). If sensation is definitely blunted or absent, tangential excision is indicated (*see* Chapter 3, pp. 87, 89), and should be scheduled for the third or fourth day after burning. In the meantime, a good dressing is applied as follows:

(i)   Wash with cetrimide–chlorhexidine solution.
(ii)   Snip blisters and remove all loose skin.
(iii)   Apply an inner layer of antiseptic tulle (e.g. Sofra-tulle) or spray with Polybactrin and apply a layer of Carbonet.
(iv)   Apply four layers of gauze, tucking in pieces of 'fluffed' gauze to separate the fingers.
(v)   Mould a plaster-of-Paris slab to the palmar surface of the hand so that the fingers are in extension at all joints. A preformed plastic splint may be used if one is available.
(vi)   Apply a layer of cotton wool.
(vii) Bandage.
(viii) Elevate the hand.

If there is doubt about the advisability of tangential excision a 'test shave' can be performed, but since this will involve what may turn out to have been an unnecessary general anaesthetic, a firm clinical decision on the ward should be taken whenever possible.

If the decision has been not to undertake tangential excision, but some delay in healing is nevertheless to be expected (e.g. if the patient's general condition is poor, or real doubt about the depth of burning persists, or the patient's cooperation is seriously in doubt), the 'plastic bag' regimen should be instituted from the outset.

The hand is cleaned, but blisters are left intact and loose skin is left *in situ*. The hand is enclosed in a voluminous plastic bag (obtainable from any supermarket) and taped at the wrist or forearm proximal to the edge of the burned area. Silver sulphadiazine cream may be applied to the burned surface before the bag is put on, but is not essential at least for the more superficial injuries (any chemical application will be toxic to the regenerating epithelial cells). The hand is then elevated and the patient encouraged to exercise the hand continuously, keeping all the joints going to the maximal extent consistent with avoidance of real discomfort. The bag is changed daily, with careful cleaning of the burned surface each time (or more frequently if the bag is damaged). Constant exercise of the digits eliminates the joint stiffness which so often follows burns of the hands which are treated too long by restrictive dressings (*see Figure 5.8*). This is a most satisfactory treatment if properly supervised; we have found it unsuitable for outpatient care, as the bag is always damaged and sepsis ensues. Closed dressings are necessary if, as frequently happens, the patients can be discharged home before epithelialization is complete. In certain circumstances the plastic bag regimen can be continued for three to four weeks, and excellent movement retained at all times.

Enclosing the burn surface in a vapour-permeable plastic sheet takes advantage of the fact that a moist 'microclimate' on the wound preserves the viability of some of the damaged exposed dermis which will die if allowed to dry out. The epithelialization occurs at a maximum rate, provided infection is avoided; this is in contrast to burns dressed conventionally by vaseline gauze and absorptive dressings, in which the surface layer of cells must die, and epithelialization must 'burrow underneath' the dead tissue, causing slower shedding of slough and more loss of skin and appendages.

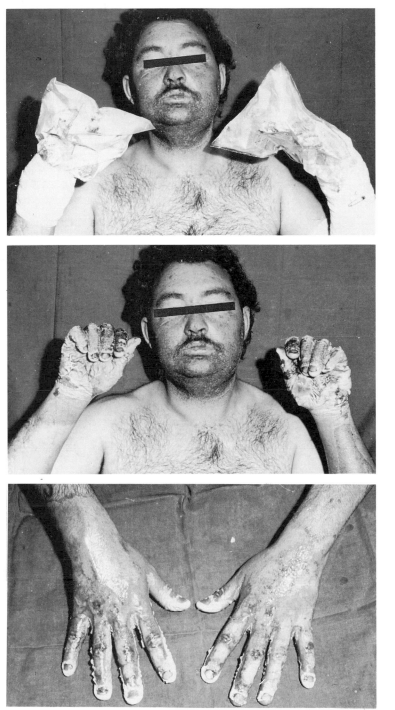

(a)

(b)

(c)

Figure 5.8 (a) Partial thickness dorsal hand burns from flash injury treated by elevation and physiotherapy while enclosed in plastic bags. (b,c) A full range of movement is preserved throughout the healing phase

Flame burns

Flame burns of mild and moderate severity have much in common with flash burns. The thin skin of the dorsum is likely to suffer more severely than the thick skin of the palm, and damage to the palms is often minimized because the hands are clenched or because they have been pressed to the face to protect the eyes at the time of the accident. These burns therefore present all the problems of the 'dorsal burn' of the hand and the treatment is the same as that described above for flash burns.

A burn of different distribution occurs when a patient tries to beat out the flames of burning clothing with his hands. The distal parts of the fingers are most severely affected, sometimes with charring of the pulps of the fingers. These patients often have extensive burns from the burning clothes. The burns of the hands are best treated conservatively with later grafting of any granulating area, and plastic bags are very useful.

Severe flame burns result from conflagrations when the patient has been trapped in a confined space and from industrial accidents involving inflammable liquids. The burns sustained by airmen in World War II were typical examples. The damage is so severe that even the thick skin of the palm is destroyed and there may be charring of the distal parts of the fingers with destruction of tendons and bones.

Treatment should be conservative in the first instance; hard circumferential eschars should be freely incised before applying the dressings, to avoid ischaemia. At a later stage, slough excision and grafting is indicated and partial amputations of fingers are often necessary. The healed hand is grossly distorted, and further reconstructive surgery is necessary.

Contact burns

Contact burns of the palm
The common type is the burn of the palm of a child who has fallen and grasped the hot element of an electric fire (Wynn Williams, 1955). These burns behave as pure heat burns and not as electrical burns (*see* Chapter 6, p. 139).

In a typical case there is no doubt about the depth of damage. The full thickness of the skin is destroyed but the neurovascular bundles and tendon sheaths are intact. The rewards of early operation in these cases are high and excellent results can be obtained by excision of the burn during the first few days and repair by thick free grafts (*Figure 5.9*). Some authorities advise a delay of four or five days before operation, on the grounds that oedema will be less by this time and there will be less danger of loss of grafts, but no real evidence has been put forward in support of this view. If full thickness skin grafting has been possible, and completely successful, further splintage after healing is not required; but if the area is extensive and thick dermatome grafts used in the primary repair, the hand should, if possible, be continuously splinted after operation until all tendency to graft shrinkage has passed (about three months). This is frequently possible for young children, but not possible (or desirable) for adults.

At the time of the first dressing, an impression of the hand is taken and an acrylic splint is constructed. The splint is applied as soon as the dressings are discarded and worn for three months, being removed only for short periods for washing of the hand, so that the graft is kept continuously on the stretch. If this is not done, some shrinkage of the graft will take place and full extension of the fingers will be lost.

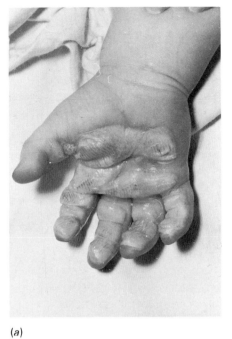

(a)

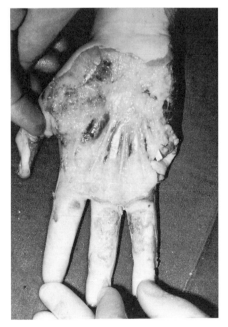

(b)

(c)

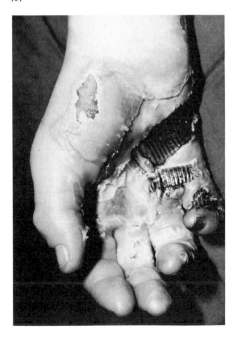

(d)

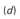

Figure 5.9

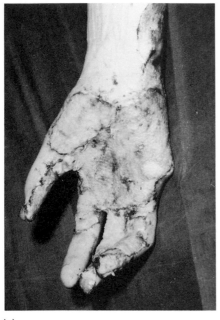

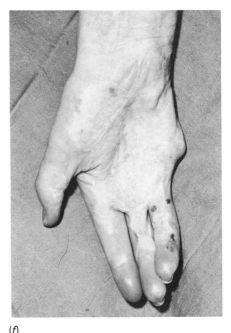

(e)   (f)

Figure 5.9 (*a*) Hand of a 1-year-old child who grasped the bar of an electric fire; (*b*) fully healed at 9 days with thick dermatome, skin grafts. No further treatment was necessary. (*c*) Burns from an electric fire sustained while the patient was drunk; (*d*) primary excision on the second day – the little finger was non-viable; (*e*) full take of split thickness skin grafts; (*f*) result at three months, with slight contracture of the thumb

If treatment has been delayed, or if there is doubt about the depth of the burn, a more conservative attitude is advisable. The burns should be treated by dressings and any granulating areas grafted with thin split-skin grafts in the usual way. These thin grafts will certainly contract and should be excised and replaced by thick grafts as a formal procedure at an early date.

In the most serious injuries of this type, not only the skin but also the tendon sheaths are destroyed. If this is the case but the tendons are intact, then repair by a pedicled flap becomes obligatory if the tendons are to be saved. The surgeon should not embark on the excisions of a deep burn of the palm unless he has sufficient experience to proceed at once to the application of an abdominal (or other suitable) flap if this proves to be necessary (*see Figure 5.10*).

Contact burns are also seen in epileptics (*see Figure 5.11*), but in these cases the distribution of the burns is more varied.

An electrical burn is a particular type of contact burn and is discussed more fully in Chapter 6.

Contact burns of the dorsum of the hand
These occur in industrial accidents due to the hand being trapped in a hot press, such as a laundry press. In the typical case, the injury is a burn of the dorsum of the hand and fingers with or without damage to the underlying tendons. The crushing

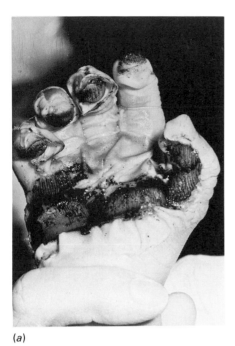

(a)

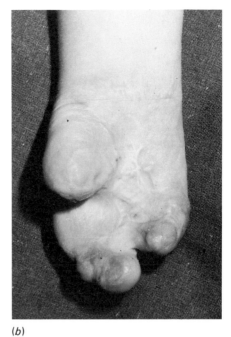

(b)

(c)

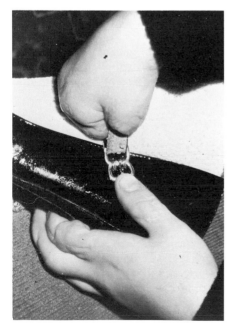

Figure 5.10 (*a*) Very severe electric fire injury at 2
years of age. (*b*) All that can be salvaged. (*c*) The
hand will retain a surprisingly good function in later
life. The patient can do up her boots at age 7 years

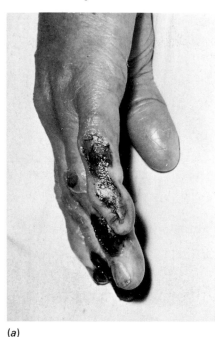

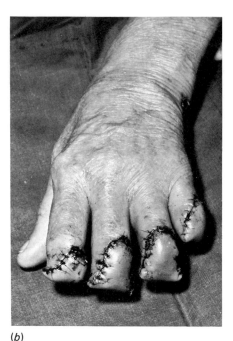

(a)   (b)

Figure 5.11 (*a*) Contact burn of the hand sustained during an epileptic attack. (*b*) Partial amputations are often necessary and are best performed early in elderly patients to preserve function in the rest of the hand

element (particularly in the common laundry press injury) is small, but in some cases crushing is more marked and there is no sharp dividing line between these and the next group – crush burns.

Some idea of the condition of the tendons can be gained at the initial examination. If the fingers are completely rigid at the metacarpophalangeal joints, then the tendons are almost certainly destroyed. Some degree of movement may still be present even when the tendons are non-viable, so that moderate degrees of damage are difficult to interpret, but free movement indicates that the tendons are viable.

If it is fairly certain from the initial examination that only the skin is involved, early excision and repair by split-skin graft is the procedure of choice.

When it seems likely from the history and examination that the tendons are involved, the treatment will differ according to the age of the patient (*see Figure 5.12*). Excision of all dead tissue usually necessitates sacrifice of the extensor tendons and sometimes of the dorsal surface of the bones as well. Cover by pedicled flap (groin flap if possible) is essential and, because elevation of the hand is then impossible, oedema is greatly prolonged and permanent stiffness is likely. This type of treatment is therefore only suitable for young supple patients. In those over 40 years and also in younger men who are thickset and whose hands are liable to become stiff, treatment should be conservative by dressings and elevation, accepting the fact that sloughing of the tendons will occur, ultimately leaving a granulating surface which can be covered with free grafts.

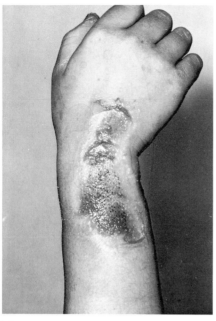
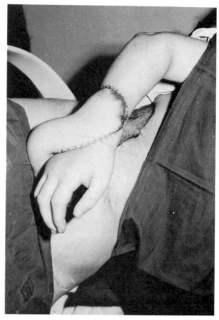

(a)   (b)

Figure 5.12 (*a*) Laundry press burns with damage to underlying tendons. (*b*) Treatment by early excision and groin flap cover. Subsequently, the flap was returned, and skin grafts applied over the salvaged tendons by this time covered with viable tissue

Crush burns

Crush burns are the result of industrial accidents and show a wide range of severity, varying from those comparable with the laundry press injuries described above, to those where the crushing element is extreme and the affected part of the hand is squashed flat and is quite dead. These severe injuries are seen after accidents in bottle and plastic moulding machines.

The treatment of moderate injuries is similar to that described for dorsal contact burns above.

If damage is very severe with squashing of the hand, amputation is usually required, using direct flaps to cover such remnants of the hand as remain.

The trunk

Burns of the trunk can often be treated by exposure, with suitable positioning of the patient. If the burn is circumferential, exposure in the early stages is still possible if the patient is treated on a turning frame, and turned every two hours. As soon as the crust becomes moist, proper dressings must be initiated, and changed every second day. Deep and extensive burns of the front of the chest, or the abdomen, sometimes cause respiratory difficulty by restricting the chest or diaphragmatic movement. In these cases, the stiff crust should be cross-hatched with a scalpel until it gapes widely and distress is relieved (*see Figure 5.13*).

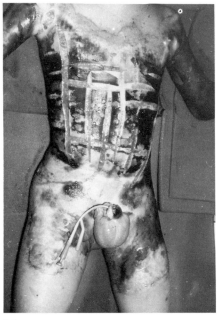

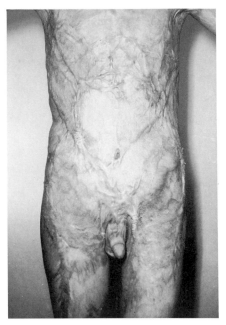

(a)   (b)

Figure 5.13 (*a*) Multiple incisions into circumferential burns of the chest to relieve life-threatening restriction of respiratory movement. (*b*) Healed burns three months later

When skin grafting is undertaken, consideration should be given to the possibility of exposing the grafts from the start (*see* Chapter 3), as movement of chest and abdomen is constant and unavoidable.

Perineum

Up to the age of five, scalds and burns of the perineum are best treated by exposure, since this is easy to achieve with the aid of a 'gallows' apparatus.

Beyond the age of five, this position is not suitable and frequent dressings with sulfamylon are best. An indwelling catheter is usually necessary in females and in males if the penis is burned; precautions against urinary sepsis must be taken (*see* Chapter 4).

Lower limbs

Thighs

Burns of the thighs may be treated by exposure if only on one surface of the limb; if circumferential, they are best wrapped up. A difficulty about extensive deep burns of the thighs is that of suitable donor sites for skin grafts, which have to be taken from the arms, trunk or lower legs (*see* Chapter 3).

Lower legs

Burns of the lower legs present no particular problem in the early stages; elevation of the feet on several pillows, or raising the foot of the bed controls oedema satisfactorily.

Difficulties often arise, however, when healing has largely been completed; not uncommonly after six weeks or so several small raw patches, about 2 cm in diameter, are all that remain unhealed, and the patient is anxious to get up. If he does so, healing will be very protracted indeed, for it seems that internal tissue pressure in the lower legs when the patient is ambulant, is sufficient to cause chronic oozing from the raw areas and thus interfere with epithelialization. Two precautions must be taken with burns of the lower legs:

(a) Healing must be complete before ambulation is attempted; it is well worth performing an extra skin grafting procedure, under local anaesthesia if desired, to obtain healing of the small discrete raw areas; an extra week in bed at this stage may save months of trouble later.

(b) A firm elastic bandage support from toes to knees is essential for at least a month after healing is complete. This bandage, if properly applied, will prevent blister formation and secondary breakdown, and will also control oedema of the foot which may be troublesome, especially in elderly people. The standard 'blue-line' one-way stretch elastic bandage is best for this purpose; crepe bandages are not satisfactory (*see Figure 5.14*).

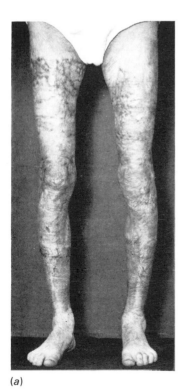

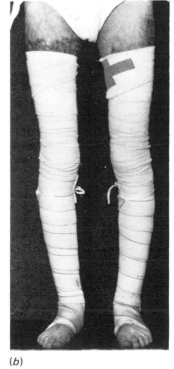

(a)   (b)

Figure 5.14 (*a*) Recently healed grafted burns of legs. (*b*) The supporting bandage

The feet

Domestic burns of the feet are not common, as the victim is usually wearing shoes or slippers when the accident occurs. Industrial burns of the feet, from molten metal, however, are very common; splashes of metal easily fall into loose boots. The depth of the burn is determined to a certain extent by the type of metal; zinc and copper alloys usually cause less damage than molten iron. The skin on the dorsum of the foot is often destroyed, the skin of the sole rarely; the dorsum offers an ideal site for primary excision and skin graft, since this can be done under tourniquet; but in practice spontaneous separation of sloughs is usually quite rapid, and little time is saved in the end by excision and graft, as opposed to secondary grafting of the granulating area. Small discrete metal burns should always be treated conservatively, being relatively painless; the patient may not need to be admitted to hospital at all, and can often continue at his work.

However, if the burns of the feet, from whatever cause, are extensive, they should always be treated in hospital, if possible, until healing is well advanced; outpatient care of such injuries almost always results in sepsis and cellulitis about 10 days after burning, and hospital admission is then urgently required and healing is delayed.

References

BRAITHWAITE, F. and WATSON, J. (1949) Some observations on the treatment of the dorsal burn of the hand. *British Journal of Plastic Surgery*, **2**, 21

GILLIES, H. (1920) *Plastic Surgery of the Face*. London: Oxford Medical Publications

HARRISON, S. H. (1952) Exposure of the skull from burns. *British Journal of Plastic Surgery*, **4**, 279

JACKSON, D. M. and STONE, P. A. (1972) Tangential excision and grafting of burns. The method and a report of 50 consecutive cases. *British Journal of Plastic Surgery*, **25**, 416–426

McINDOE, SIR A. H. (1983) Total Reconstruction of the Burned Face. Bradshaw Lecture 1958. *British Journal of Plastic Surgery*, **36**, 410–420

ROBERTS, A. H. N. (1983) The preservation of hair in burns of the scalp. *Plastic and Reconstructive Surgery*, **72**, 869–871

SCHOFIELD, A. L. (1954) A review of burns of the eyelids and their treatment. *British Journal of Plastic Surgery*, **4**, 113

WYNN WILLIAMS, D. (1955) A review of burned hands in children. *British Journal of Plastic Surgery*, **7**, 313

Chapter 6

Burns of special types

Although most burns are due to thermal trauma, burns due to other agencies are not uncommon. Many of the remarks which apply to heat burns apply also to burns due to other causes, but some have specific features which alter the prognosis and make modifications of treatment essential.

The types of burns to be considered are:

(1) Electrical burns.
(2) Chemical burns.
(3) Burns due to hot metal.
(4) Burns due to radioactive emanations.

Electrical burns

The majority of electrical burns are due to contact with the domestic electrical supply (220–240 volts AC); burns caused by contact with the high voltage grid system (11 000–66 000 volts AC) are occasionally seen.

The following clinical conditions should be considered:

Burns due to electric flash without actual contact   The damage is usually superficial, although the hand or face is sometimes covered in a black film of volatized metal which gives it an alarming appearance. When the film is removed the skin is found to be almost undamaged.

Hot element burns (i.e. sustained on the red-hot element of an electric fire)   These are pure heat burns, and behave as such; they are almost always full thickness, as contact is prolonged by reason of spasm of the hand muscles. They are often suitable for early excision and grafting, but loss of part or all of digits is unfortunately a common sequel of the more severe injuries (*see* Chapter 5, pp. 138–140).

Arcing injuries   These are uncommon and tend to give rise to localized deep burns.

Lightning burns   These have an irregular branched appearance and may involve full-thickness loss. General effects are severe (Arden *et al.*, 1956).

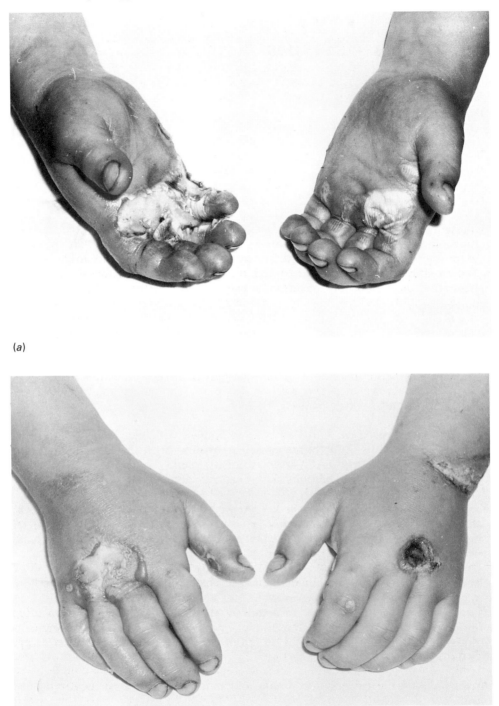

(a)

(b)

Figure 6.1 (*a*) Extensive domestic current electrical fire burn from a faulty electric fire. (*b*) Dorsal exit burns

True electrical burns – contact burns (Muir, 1971)   The damage is due to passage of electricity through the tissues, and the amount of destruction depends on the strength of the current (in amperes) and the time during which contact is maintained. The strength of the current depends partly on the nature of the supply (in volts) and the nature of the contact with the skin (i.e. the resistance). Firm contact with wet skin will allow more current to pass than light contact with dry skin.

The natural history of these injuries differs so much from that of thermal injuries that it is clear that the electric current has some specific effect and the damage is not due solely to the heating effect of the passage of the current.

There is always an entry and an exit burn, but because of differences in contact they may differ greatly in severity (*Figure 6.1*).

The skin component of an electrical burn is clearly demarcated, and corresponds with the area of contact. Deep to the skin, the damage decreases with increasing depth. Because of their fluid content blood vessels form good conductors, and thrombosis of digital or other vessels may occur with serious consequences.

In a heat burn the dividing line between dead and surviving tissue soon becomes clearcut, and a healthy zone of reaction develops in the surviving tissue. The slough separates in 14–21 days exposing red healthy granulations, on which skin grafts take readily. In an electrical burn, however, the healing reaction in the marginal zone of surviving tissue is imperfect and slow to develop. The sloughs separate slowly, exposing pale oedematous granulations on which skin grafts will not take. Furthermore, the surviving but damaged tissue by reason of its depressed cellular activity, offers poor resistance to bacterial invasion, and infection may lead to progressive necrosis of tissue with exposure of tendons or joints which were previously thought to be out of danger.

Clinical features

Electrical burns occur most commonly on the hands (*see Figure 6.1*).

The horny layer of skin is raised and loose. When this loose skin is removed, the area of skin destruction is seen as a dead white area with a narrow surrounding rim of bright red. The necrotic skin becomes black, and separates after many weeks, disclosing pale lilac-coloured granulations. Final healing is slow.

In more severe burns separation of sloughs results in exposure of tendons, bones or joints, and sloughing of tendon or sequestration of bone and cartilage may follow.

In domestic supply accidents, although the burn may be deep, the area of deep damage corresponds approximately with the area of superficial damage, and extension under intact skin is limited. Occasionally main vessels underlying the burn are damaged and become thrombosed, resulting in gangrene in the part distal to the burn. With this exception, the area of skin destruction remains confined to its original dimensions, and does not extend.

In high tension injuries, the current gains entrance through the skin and passes up the centre of the limb as it would up the core of a conducting cable, causing extensive necrosis of vessels, muscles and nerves. Gangrene due to vascular insufficiency often occurs.

Treatment

Domestic supply injuries
Except in very minor injuries the skin is destroyed in its full thickness, and early excision and repair should be carried out.

Early operation has been criticized on the grounds that, when free grafts are used, the grafts are often lost and there is progressive necrosis of tissue previously thought to be healthy. This occurs because the tissue, although initially alive, is not healthy enough to take grafts and, when the grafts fail to take, is exposed to the danger of infection.

If excision of the burn is followed by the application of a healthy flap bearing its own blood supply, infection does not occur and good healing is obtained (Muir, 1958).

The recommended treatment is therefore:

(1) Early excision of the burn back to healthy tissue. It is particularly important that the edge of the burn, where a small rim of partial thickness damage is invariably present, should be included in the excision, otherwise the flap repair will not adhere properly.
(2) Repair by local flap (e.g. cross-finger flap) if possible, otherwise by distant flap. The fasciocutaneous flap (*see* Chapter 5) is particularly recommended for cross-forearm use in this situation, as its excellent blood supply enables a long pedicle to be incorporated in the design, so that movements in the undamaged fingers can be encouraged throughout the period of immobilization.
(3) Repair by free graft only if it is certain that the burn is relatively superficial, and if no important structures will be endangered should the graft fail.

No surgeon should embark on the excision of an electrical burn unless he is able and prepared to perform a flap repair on the spot.

High tension injuries
These present great difficulties in management. Excision of damaged tissue and repair by flap is theoretically the ideal treatment, but in practice this is a course of such magnitude and difficulty that a more conservative attitude is usually adopted.

Amputations are often necessary (*see Figure 6.2*).

General effects

Unconsciousness and death often occur with electrical injuries. Unconsciousness is frequently associated with paralysis of respiration, and artificial respiration should be commenced at once.

In other instances, ventricular fibrillation occurs, and although this has been treated in experimental animals by means of an electrical defibrillator, there is no record of its having been used in man. External cardiac massage, properly conducted, has a good chance of success and should be instituted immediately.

Shock occurs only in severe high-tension injuries, and in association with severe muscle damage. It should be treated on the same lines as shock due to physical trauma, with whole blood as the main fluid for transfusion.

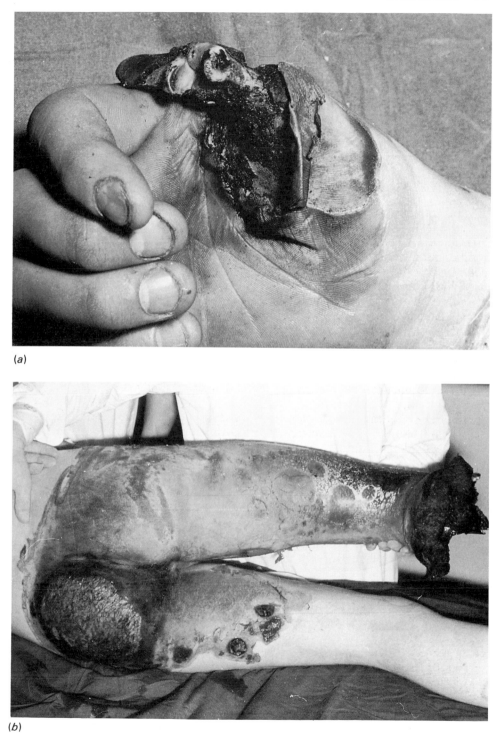

(a)

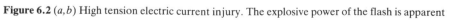

(b)

Figure 6.2 (*a,b*) High tension electric current injury. The explosive power of the flash is apparent

Chemical burns

These usually occur in industrial accidents and in laboratories. Burns due to phosphorus from incendiary bombs were seen in wartime, as might also be burns due to irritant gases such as mustard gas.

The substances most likely to be encountered are:

(*a*) Acid – sulphuric, hydrochloric, nitric, hydrofluoric.
(*b*) Alkali – caustic soda (sodium hydroxide), caustic potash (potassium hydroxide), lime (calcium oxide).
(*c*) Phenols – phenol, lysol.
(*d*) Phosphorus.

Immediate treatment

The immediate treatment of all chemical burns is to remove the active substance as soon as possible by washing the affected part under running water. This should be done before any search for an antidote is made. The only exception is with burns from lime, where any solid should be removed before washing is begun. When washing has removed as much of the chemical as possible, an antidote may be applied if one is available.

For acids – sodium bicarbonate.
For alkalis – vinegar, ammonium chloride.

Acid and alkali burns are often deep and, particularly with alkali, the chemical may penetrate deeply into the tissue and continue to cause damage, even when the excess surface chemical has been removed. An obviously full thickness alkali burn should therefore be treated by early excision, and the pH of the underlying tissue determined at operation. If this is high, then dressings of vinegar should be applied and grafting delayed until the area is obviously healthy.

Hydrofluoric acid burns

Hydrofluoric acid is widely used in glass manufacture, pottery, glazing, in the electronics industry and as a cleaning agent for toilet walls and surrounds and granite surfaces. Contact with the skin results in a burn (Goodfellow, 1985) which has special characteristics.

(1) It is accompanied by intense pain.
(2) The skin is coagulated.
(3) Progressive destruction of deeper tissues occurs in the absence of treatment.
(4) The burn frequently extends subungually, and access for topical applications is restricted.

The initial appearance is of erythema only, but coagulation and progressive destruction of tissue are common in the absence of treatment. Goodfellow, from an experience of over 600 cases, recommends as follows:

(1) Immediate flushing with cold water at the scene of the accident for 20 min.
(2) Application of iced water until the pain subsides. An extensive trial of calcium gluconate gel revealed much less effective pain control, and no discernible

difference in healing. Iced water applications were much preferred by those patients who had experience of both treatments.

However, calcium gluconate can be brought to the site of damaged but viable tissue by injecting a solution intravenously into a hand or forearm vein with the circulation arrested by a pneumatic tourniquet, in the same way as local anaesthetic is injected in the Bier block procedure. In these injuries the tourniquet can usually be placed on the forearm; 5 ml of 10 per cent calcium gluconate should be injected and the tourniquet retained for 10 min. In the few patients who have been treated by this method, pain relief has been rapid and it has not been necessary to repeat the injection.

(3) Removal of the nail if the acid has penetrated beneath it.
(4) Cover of the burned area with dressings or medicaments for small areas until healing occurs.
(5) Excision of the burn with immediate skin grafting is the treatment of choice if the area is large enough to warrant it.

Phenol burns

Phenol penetrates deeply into the skin and, unless the chemical is removed quickly enough, may be absorbed to give systemic and local effects. The phenol will continue to penetrate deeply causing further damage, and enough may be absorbed to cause toxic effects, of which kidney damage is the most important.

For these reasons early excision should always be considered.

Phosphorus burns

These have been caused by incendiary bombs. Particles of elemental phosphorus are liable to be driven into the tissues and will continue to cause damage until washed or picked out. The wound should be flooded with a 1 per cent copper sulphate solution which will turn the phosphorus particles black and facilitate identification.

For extensive phosphorus injuries, Ben Hur *et al.* (1972) recommend 5 per cent bicarbonate + 1 per cent hydroxyethylcellulose + 3 per cent copper sulphate, as absorption of large amounts of copper sulphate can cause severe renal damage.

Hot metal burns

Burns due to molten metal occur in men working in foundries.

In the typical injury the molten metal is splashed or spilled onto the legs and some of it may run down inside the boots, causing burns of the feet. In some cases there are small scattered burns and this type of injury heals well under conservative treatment.

In other instances, the burns are confluent, with well-defined edges, and early excision should be considered if the full thickness of the skin is obviously destroyed. This is usually easy to determine when the thin skin of the dorsum of the foot is involved, but in the thick skin of the sole it may be difficult. In the latter instance, a conservative policy is indicated because no skin graft is ever a complete substitute for the specialized sole skin. In spite of this, if sole skin is destroyed, the results of repair by split-skin graft are good, as long as an adequate depth of the specialized subcutaneous tissue of the sole remains intact.

Burns due to radioactive emanations

Radiation burns

These may be seen in the acute or chronic stages. They may be due to excessive doses during radiotherapy, or radiodiagnosis or to accidents involving nuclear energy apparatus.

Acute phase
Within one or two days of the irradiation the affected area becomes red and swollen and may blister. In most instances the burn is of partial thickness depth and heals slowly over the course of a few months.

Chronic phase
The healed post-irradiated skin is always abnormal to a greater or lesser degree. In a typical case it is atrophic, hairless, indurated and white with red spidery telangiectases. This atrophic skin may later break down, forming a simple ulcer, or undergo malignant change and become a squamous-celled carcinoma.

In other instances where the initial damage is less acute, the early changes may be mild and transient, but chronic changes appear months or years later. In the most severe forms of radiation damage, destruction may be so severe that healing never occurs.

Treatment
Acute stage   Treatment is conservative by means of soothing applications to allay irritation.

Chronic stage   Treatment will certainly be necessary for ulceration or malignant change, and may be undertaken in earlier non-ulcerated lesions as a prophylactic measure, because of itching and irritation or for cosmetic reasons.

Treatment is by excision of the irradiated skin and repair of the defect. Free grafts take poorly on irradiated tissue and can only be used if the damage is fairly superficial. In most cases, repair must be by means of a flap bearing its own blood supply. If the surrounding tissue is healthy it may be possible to make use of a local flap, but more often it will be necessary to import tissue from a distance by means of an open flap or a tubed pedicle. Flaps nourished by free microvascular anastomosis can also be very useful if the nearby arteries and veins are intact, and can eliminate the necessity for awkward immobilizations in elderly patients.

Burns due to nuclear explosions

Information about these injuries has come from studies of the atomic bomb explosions at Hiroshima and Nagasaki in 1945, and from various test explosions. Some animal laboratory experiments also bear on this problem.

After the atomic bomb explosions in 1945, the majority of the survivors had burns due to exposure to the intense heat flash. Other burns were caused by fires started by the flash (Oughterson and Warren, 1956).

Actual burns due to nuclear radiations (neutrons, gamma-rays and X-rays) did not occur, presumably because anyone close enough to the centre of the explosion to receive a sufficient skin dose to cause a burn would have received a fatal dose of irradiation or was killed by heat, although the occurrence of epilation indicated that there was some specific skin damage.

The general effects of whole-body irradiation were manifest in two ways:

(1) If the dosage was sufficiently high the specific effects of radiation sickness appeared – nausea, vomiting, diarrhoea, ulceration of mucous membranes, haemorrhage.
(2) The morbidity and mortality of patients with thermal burns was greater in irradiated than in non-irradiated patients. The evidence indicates, and has been confirmed by laboratory studies, that morbidity and mortality of thermal burns is increased even when the irradiation dose is below that required to cause specific clinical effects.

The desirable treatments for heat burns after an atomic explosion do not differ from those used for burns of different causation, but administrative requirements would certainly modify the treatment available. Further aspects are discussed in Chapter 9.

Effects due to radioactive fall-out were not noted after the 1945 explosions, but were seen in the crew of the Japanese fishing vessel Lucky Dragon, which was accidentally contaminated by radioactive dust from a test H-bomb explosion at Bikini Atoll in 1954. The crew suffered from the general effects of radiation sickness and also from subacute radiation burns from lodgement of radioactive dust in the skin.

Details of the number of patients, type and degree of illness and treatment given following the Chernobyl nuclear power station explosion (April, 1986) remain to be published.

Further reading and references

ARDEN, G. P., HARRISON, S. H., LISTER, J. and MAUDSLEY, R. H. (1956) Lightning accident at Ascot. *British Medical Journal*, **1**, 1450

BEN HUR, N., GILADY, A., APPELBAUM, J. and NEUMAN, Z. (1972) Phosphorus burns; the antidote: a new approach. *British Journal of Plastic Surgery*, **25**, 245

CRAIG, R. D. P. (1964) Hydrofluoric acid burns of the hands. *British Journal of Plastic Surgery*, **17**, 63

GOODFELLOW, R. C. (1985) Hydrofluoric acid burns. *British Medical Journal*, **290**, 937

MUIR, I. F. K. (1958) The treatment of electrical burns. *British Journal of Plastic Surgery*, **10**, 292

MUIR, I. F. K. (1971) Treatment of electrical burns. In *Transactions of the Fifth International Congress of Plastic and Reconstructive Surgery*, p. 862. Sydney: Butterworths

OUGHTERSON, A. W. and WARREN, S. (1956) *Medical Effects of the Atomic Bomb in Japan*. New York: McGraw-Hill

Chapter 7

First aid and rescue
out-patient treatment of minor burns

First aid

Under this heading are included the rescue procedures to be carried out in burning accidents, and also the preliminary help given to an injured person before arrival of the doctor.

Rescue

Prompt action is vital.

Victim in burning room   The victim may be unconscious from poisoning by carbon monoxide or inhalation or smoke or, if a child, may be too terrified to find the way out of the room. The rescuer should cover his nose and mouth with a handkerchief soaked in water, and crawl along the floor of the room, where the smoke is likely to be least dense. He should pull the victim to safety, and if necessary immediately apply mouth-to-mouth artificial respiration.

Victim with clothes on fire   The victim should be laid down and the flames smothered with a rug or coat.

Victim scalded with hot fluid   The clothes, which probably still contain hot fluid, should be removed immediately.

Electric shock   If possible the current should be switched off. If this is impossible the victim must be removed from contact with the live conductor. The body must not be touched with bare hands. The person can either be pulled away by seizing his clothes, or be pushed off with a dry wooden handle or stick. If the victim is not breathing, mouth-to-mouth respiration should be instituted and, if there is no pulse, external cardiac massage should be started. If these measures are carried out promptly, many electrocuted victims will survive.

Acute care of the burn

Any clothes which can be easily removed should be, but particles of clothing which are adherent to the skin should not be pulled off roughly.

There is no doubt that for minor burns the most satisfactory method of immediate treatment is to place the part under cold running water and keep it there for some minutes. Not only does this relieve pain, but it in no way interferes with the subsequent examination of the injury. (By contrast, application of such substances as butter or acriflavine emulsion may confuse the picture.)

Whether it is wise to advocate that extensive burns should be treated in a similar manner is doubtful. In view of the known dangers of delay in instituting fluid therapy for shock in severe burns, the bystanders should certainly telephone for an ambulance before considering local applications for the burn itself. On the other hand, there is clear experimental evidence that immediate cooling of the burned part can minimize tissue damage and, if a good supply of clean cold water is immediately to hand it would seem sensible to use it, provided that help is *on the way*.

Application of 'coolpaks' to the burned surface has everything to recommend it, both to decrease the amount of pain and in the hope of minimizing tissue damage, and supplies of these might be made available both in the ambulance and the casualty department as a routine.

Assessment

Under peace-time conditions, in countries with well-developed hospital services, any patient who has sustained a burn of more than 5 per cent of the body surface should be admitted to hospital. If hospital treatment is indicated the burn should be covered with a sterile dressing if such is available; alternatively a clean sheet or towel can be used, and urgent transport to hospital arranged.

Transport

From the site of the accident, transport should obviously be by the swiftest means practicable to the nearest hospital casualty department. But care must be taken to avoid any additional trauma.

It frequently happens, in the case of serious burns, that a further journey to a specialist department, either a plastic surgery centre or a burns centre, is required during the first few hours after injury. It should be remembered that, however careful the driver, an ambulance journey is accompanied by a considerable amount of vibration and even jolting, especially in heavy traffic. It is therefore essential that any transfusion on the journey must be trouble-free, since it will often be impossible for the attendant to tell whether the drip is still running, let alone giving the correct rate per minute. A needle in a vein will almost always migrate under these conditions and, if the transfusion gets behind-hand, leg veins will go into spasm. We most strongly recommend, therefore, that a cannula be used, preferably introduced by cut-down, and that an arm vein be selected. It is true to say that, whenever a leg vein has been used in patients arriving at the Pinderfields Burns Centre, over the last 20 years, the transfusion stopped either before or shortly after admission, and had to be re-erected elsewhere. Clearly lives can be jeopardized if precautions are not observed.

Selection of patients for non-hospital care

The following general rules should be borne in mind when deciding if the patient can be treated on a domiciliary basis:

(1) The burn should be inspected in a good light and its extent and depth estimated. The history is often helpful: if the injury is a scald, was the fluid boiling or merely hot? If the injury is a burn, was the contact momentary or prolonged?

(2) These burns, even if of small extent, are not suitable for treatment at home:

   (a) Well-defined deep burns on any part of the body where early excision and grafting may be indicated.

   (b) Burns of the face or hands, if there is any suspicion that part of the burn may be deep. If there is doubt about the depth, the hospital surgeon will prefer to supervise the care from the outset, so that he can proceed to grafting without delay if this should prove necessary.

   (c) Burns in areas such as the perineum, which are awkward to manage.

(3) Many burns are better suited to home care than to hospital management, the patient nearly always preferring to remain at home if possible. These include:

   (a) Obviously superficial burns on any part of the body.

   (b) Burns of mixed or doubtful depth on areas other than face or hands. If it seems likely that there may be some full-thickness loss, there should be no hesitation in obtaining a surgical opinion either at home or in the out-patient department, but even if the burn is deep the best course may well be to continue with out-patient care until the area is ready for grafting.

Dressing technique

(1) Wash gently with cetrimide–chlorhexidine solution.

(2) Remove all completely loose skin. Unless the blisters are very large, they should be left. Large blisters which look as though they may burst may be punctured and the contents evacuated, but the overlying skin should be left to protect the raw area underneath.

(3) Apply two layers of Bactigras or similar non-adherent dressing.

(4) Apply four layers of gauze.

(5) Apply a layer of cotton-wool, making sure that it extends for four inches over normal skin on all sides of the burn.

(6) Bandage carefully, so that all parts of the dressing are covered, and the edges will not slip.

The second dressing

This should be done on the fourth day after the injury. The bandage, wool, gauze and one layer of tulle are removed, leaving the second layer in place. Further gauze and cotton-wool are applied without any washing or cleaning, and may be less bulky than before. A careful reapplication of the bandage, if clean, or a fresh bandage, completes the procedure.

Third dressing

This is performed after another seven days have elapsed. Many superficial burns will be found to have healed at this time. If the wound is not yet healed, but is obviously healing, another dressing is applied for a further few days; if there is any full thickness slough, or if infection has supervened, the treatment should be changed to frequent wet dressings with eusol.

Eusol dressings

These dressings should be done at least once a day, and the gauze soaked in eusol applied directly to the wound without any intervening tulle (*see* p. 176).

At each dressing, the previously applied gauze should be soaked off to minimize pain and to avoid pulling off new epithelium.

Grafting

Any raw area greater than an inch in diameter should be grated, and small areas can be satisfactorily dealt with in the casualty department under local or general anaesthesia. Patients with larger areas to be covered will need admission to hospital for a short time.

Antibiotics

There is usually no indication for the administration of systemic antibiotics to patients with burns suitable for out-patient treatment. If infection should occur, this is almost always the result of faulty dressing technique, or interference with the dressing by the patient or his relatives; and in these circumstances it will be best to refer the patient to hospital. In the great majority of cases, no infection occurs at any stage when the injury is properly treated at home.

Further reading

WALLACE, A. B. (1961) First aid treatment of burns and scalds. *Practitioner*, **187**, 16

Chapter 8

Scars and contractures

The degree of scarring left by a burn depends on the depth and site of the burn and the age of the patient.

In superficial partial thickness burns, the healed skin is of good texture and elasticity; at first there may be some depigmentation of the area, but this gradually returns to normal.

All deep partial thickness burns result in scarring, and in full thickness burns scars form at the margins of grafts and in areas which have healed by secondary epithelialization. Burns scars, like all other scars, go through a series of phases, being initially flat and fairly inconspicuous, then red, thick and hard, and finally flat, white and soft.

Hypertrophic scars

In many burns scars, the phase of redness and hardness is excessive both in intensity and duration and the condition is then termed 'hypertrophic scar'.

In deep partial thickness burns hypertrophic scarring is so common that it may be considered normal. The hypertrophy reaches its maximum intensity about three months after healing, the scar then remains static for a period and gradually resolves over the course of one to two years, becoming pale, softer and flatter. During the active phase the scar is often intensely itchy.

It cannot be too strongly emphasized that the course described above is a common and normal sequence and that spontaneous resolution can be confidently predicted. Considerable symptomatic relief can be afforded to patients with hypertrophic scars, and pressure garment therapy can minimize the degree of hypertrophy and speed resolution, but there is little evidence that the final result can be influenced by any form of treatment (*Figure 8.1*). In particular it should be noted that any surgical treatment at this stage is almost certain to be followed by further hypertrophic scarring and, unless there are specially urgent reasons, surgery should be delayed until the stage of hypertrophy has passed.

It is important, however, that any patient who has a deep partial thickness or full thickness burn should be kept under observation for at least three months after healing, so that the development of hypertrophic scarring can be observed and the patient suitably and promptly advised. If this is not done the patient may think that something has gone wrong and blame the surgeon.

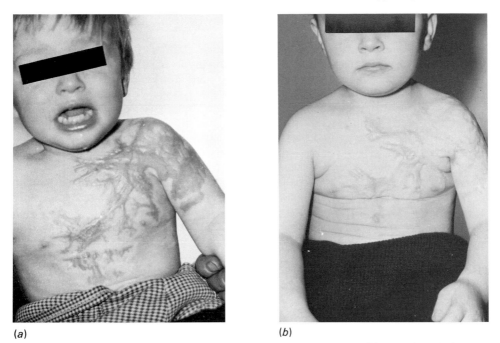

(a)   (b)

Figure 8.1 (*a*) Itchy scars from an extensive scald cause considerable distress. (*b*) Natural resolution after one year

Radiotherapy has been used for this condition. It is believed that there is no evidence that radiotherapy has any beneficial effect on established hypertrophic scars. This powerful weapon should be kept in reserve and may in selected cases be of use in preventing further hypertrophic scarring after elective surgical correction of residual scars (Mowlem, 1952).

It is important that these hypertrophic scars (which are common) are not confused with true keloids (which are very rare). The natural history of keloids is quite different, inasmuch as they do not tend to resolve after a few months but continue to grow for many months and years, and appear to invade normal tissue beyond the confines of the original scar. A burn is no more likely to be followed by a keloid than is any other injury.

Treatment

Hypertrophic scars should be treated conservatively. The main disability, apart from the unsightly appearance, is the itching which may be very distressing; severe pruritus is commonest in young children and worse in bed, where the surroundings are warm. The parents are often distracted because the child cannot get to sleep and the child himself may lose weight and be out of sorts during the irritable phase.

Treatment is difficult, but may be on the following lines:

(1) *Reassurance* The parents, and the patient if old enough, must be convinced that this is a passing phase, inevitable because of the nature of the injury, and that complete relief from irritation is certain with the lapse of time. Having made sure that this is understood:

(2) *Antipuritic ointments or lotions*   These may be tried, such as calamine with 1 per cent phenol or camphor.

(3) *Steroid applications*   Some success has been claimed for treatment by local applications of steroids such as 1 per cent hydrocortisone or triamcinolone either in ointments or creams or in impregnated adhesive tape, but the results are often disappointing. Steroid injections which are sometimes suitable for small hypertrophies scars are not suitable for extensive burns scars.

(4) *Massage*   It is doubtful if local massage has more than a minimal effect in hastening resolution of the hypertrophic scar. Nevertheless, massage with a bland cream gives comfort, and the patient may feel more satisfied that something active is being done. It should be made clear, however, that the local massage must be done by patient or parents, and not by the physiotherapy department. The best application is probably simple lanoline cream, which should be made up to a soft consistency as follows:

Anhydrous lanoline	6 parts
Liquid paraffin	1 part
Arachis oil	1 part

(5) *Systemic antihistamines*   If sleep is being disturbed by itching, systemic antihistamines should be tried. It is not clear if these have any specific effects or if they merely act as hypnotics.

(6) *Pressure*   The work of Larson and his colleagues (1971) has shown that hypertrophic scars can be prevented or treated with the application of continuous pressure and this is confirmed from the authors own practice. This is not difficult to achieve for scars of the legs and feet, less easy for the hands and arms, and very difficult for the trunk and face, although Larson is so convinced of the value of this treatment that he makes up close-fitting masks so that evenly distributed pressure can be achieved, even on the face. The garments are expensive, and therapy needs to be continued for at least 12 months. During this time, four or more new garments will be required, as the old ones lose their elasticity, and patient (or parent) compliance is sometimes not easily achieved. It is our belief that many more garments are prescribed than are actually worn, and this potentially valuable but costly treatment should be reserved for those patients who both really need it and have parents to whom the requirements can be explained with a full sympathetic understanding of the problems involved.

Keloid scars

True keloid scars are extremely difficult to treat, but are fortunately very rare. Excision followed by the long continued wearing of close-fitting pressure moulds are the best hope, but even this treatment may be very disappointing.

Secondary surgery for appearance

Even in the absence of contracture, the appearance of an old burn scar or a patchwork of skin graft and junctional scar may be sufficiently unsightly for plastic surgery to be undertaken (*Figure 8.2*). Since this surgery will almost invariably

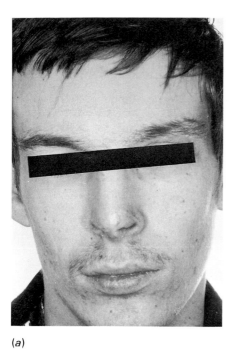

(a)

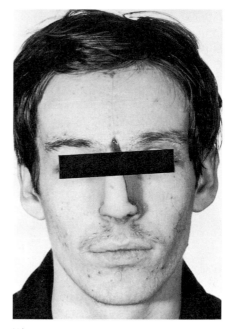

(b)

(c)

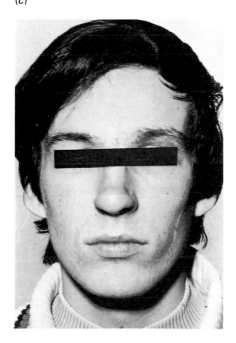

Figure 8.2 (a) Loss of tip of the nose due to contact
burn in childhood. (b) Forehead flap repair.
(c) Early result

involve extensive skin grafting, with the accompanying discomfort, the patient himself will often be the best judge of whether the effort will be worthwhile. The appearance of a skin graft, however good the take, is abnormal because of skin colour differences and lack of hair growth, and these factors must be taken into account when deciding about surgery for appearance. As stated above, the hypertrophic phase of scar maturation must be over before surgery is embarked on. When improvement in appearance is the sole objective, better results are usually obtained by shaving the surface until it is level with the surrounding skin and applying a thin skin graft rather than excising the whole thickness of the scar and applying thick grafts, which take with more difficulty and often remain permanently too pale. This tangential excision is best carried out freehand with a No. 22 blade unless the area is very extensive, in which case the use of a guarded skin graft knife is more appropriate and less time consuming.

Contractures

All scars and free grafts tend to shrink; thin grafts shrink more than thick ones. Contractures are, therefore, common sequelae to severe burns and late reconstructive procedures are often necessary.

Most joints readily assume a position of flexion; grafts and scars on flexor aspects are not naturally subjected to tension and, therefore, shrink markedly. Over the extensor aspects of joints, grafts and scars are constantly put on the stretch by the powerful flexor muscles and shrinkage is therefore minimal.

This process of shrinkage is associated with the maturation of the scar tissue and bears a relation in time to the redness and thickness of the scar. The shrinkage (like the state of hypertrophy of the scar) is maximal at three months and thereafter some slight relaxation of the scar may take place.

Early contractures

A mild early contracture may sometimes be relieved naturally over a period of a few months by stretching and migration of surrounding tissues. If this is thought probable, an expectant policy is justifiable provided that the patient attends at regular intervals so that surgery can be undertaken if the contracture does not improve.

It is sometimes possible, in children, to immobilize a part which has been recently skin grafted, in such a position that the graft is constantly on the stretch until the tendency to shrink has passed – usually about three months. For this prolonged immobilization to be justifiable, the graft must be of adequate thickness so that after three months of immobilization the splint can be discarded and no further surgery is required. The parts where this technique is of most use are the elbow and the flexor aspects of the fingers. The necessary position must be maintained by an accurately fitting plaster cast or moulded splint. The technique is not suitable for adults because of the danger of permanent joint stiffness.

Larson *et al.* (1971) have demonstrated dramatic effects, even in severe early contracture, by traction and serial splintage.

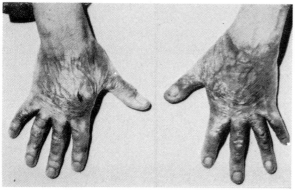

(a)

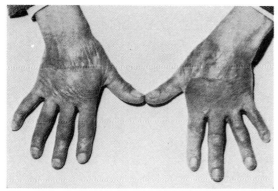

(b)

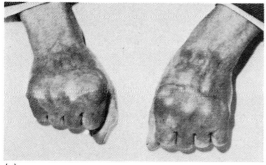

(c)

Figure 8.3 (*a*) Scarring of dorsum of hands. Notice cracks due to stretching of unstable scars. There was limitation of flexion of the metacarpophalangeal joints. (*b*) The scars have been excised and replaced by thick split-skin grafts taken from the abdomen by a Padgett dermatome. (*c*) Good flexion is restored

Limitation of joint movement

Skin contractures may cause limitation of joint movement. As long as the joint capsule remains healthy, release of the skin contracture will result in the restoration of joint movement.

In some situations, however, if joint excursion is severely limited for a prolonged period by skin contracture, secondary shrinkage of the joint capsule occurs and joint mobility will not be regained even when the skin deformity is corrected. This condition is particularly likely to arise in the metacarpophalangeal joints of the hand following burns of the dorsum with subsequent skin shortage, and also in flexion contracture of the proximal interphalangeal joints following burns of the flexor aspect of the fingers (*see Figures 8.3* and *8.4* and Chapter 5).

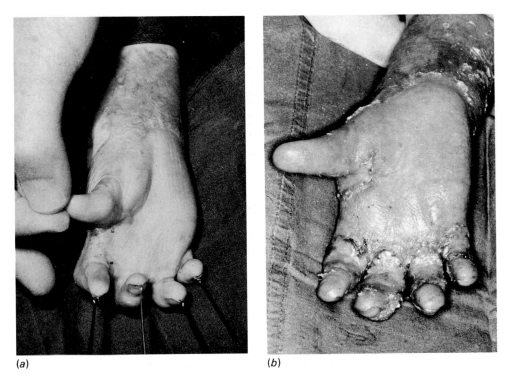

(a)   (b)

Figure 8.4 (*a*) Established contracture of all fingers and thumb due to volar skin destruction. (*b*) Contracture released with full thickness skin grafts

Even in the absence of skin loss, limitation of joint excursion can sometimes occur because of capsular changes due to immobilization in a faulty position. This is liable to happen in the ankle joints, which easily become stiff in plantar flexion, and also in the metacarpophalangeal joints of the fingers; it is important that these conditions should not be confused with limitation of joint mobility due to scar contracture.

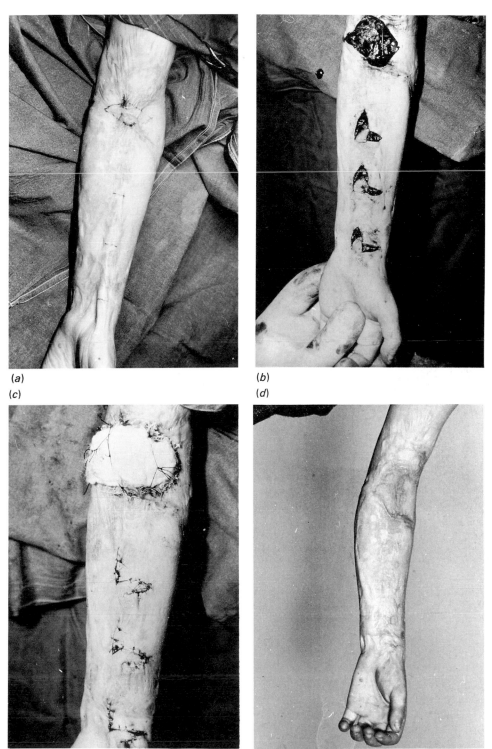

(a)

(b)

(c)

(d)

Figure 8.5 (*a*) Contracture on flexor surface of the elbow, with subsidiary linear band of scar on the distal forearm. (*b*) Release by multiple cross-cuts. (*c*) Repair by skin graft to elbow and fasciocutaneous transposed flaps to forearm. (*d*) Result at three months

Established contractures

Established contractures which interfere with function must be relieved. Three surgical methods are available:

(1) Local rearrangement of the skin.
(2) Free grafting.
(3) Pedicled flap transfer.

Local arrangement of skin

This is accomplished by single or multiple Z-plasties or small skin flaps transposed through a right angle. It used to be thought that only undamaged skin adjacent to a contracture had a sufficiently good blood supply to withstand such rearrangement, but it has recently been shown that small random flaps raised in scarred tissue or old skin graft retain their viability provided the deep fascia is raised with the flap (Barclay, 1986). Provided that there is sufficient laxity in a transverse direction, transposition of multiple small flaps provides excellent permanent release of scarred bands or grooves without secondary skin grafting being necessary (*Figure 8.5*). In general, transposed flaps are best for raised bands, and Z-plasties for grooves (*Figure 8.6*).

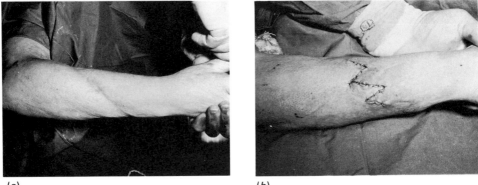

(a)   (b)

Figure 8.6 (*a*) Groove on the extensor aspect of the forearm. (*b*) Release by multiple fasciocutaneous Z-plasties

Free grafting

For all except linear contractures, addition of skin in both longitudinal and transverse directions is required. Adequate release is achieved by cross cut right out into normal tissue, and thick split-skin grafting will usually provide a sufficiently permanent correction (if the scarred area is small, excision rather than incision may be best). Notoriously the front of the neck will require more than one release as the new skin graft shrinks in its turn.

Repair by pedicled skin flap

The advantage of skin transferred by pedicled flap is that it shows no tendency to shrink when transfer is complete.

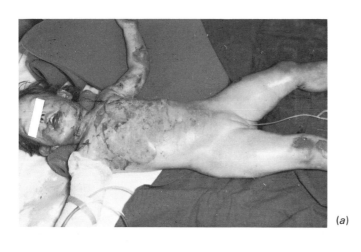

(a)

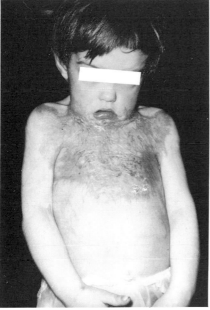

(b)

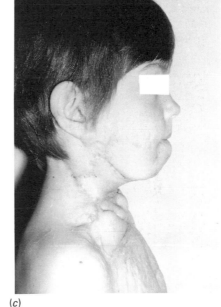

(c)

Figue 8.7 (*a*) Full thickness burn of the chest, neck and lower face from burning nightdress. (*b*) Gross contracture despite skin grafting. (*c*) Repair by tubed pedicle skin flap

Disadvantages of the method are that it requires many operations to complete the repair, is very time consuming, and leaves extensive scarring at the donor site. For these reasons it is normally reserved for areas where free grafts give unsatisfactory results (e.g. front of neck), or where surgery on the joints themselves is contemplated and good cover is essential (*see Figure 8.7*).

Microvascular surgery can overcome some of these snags and reduce the number of operations required; but even in the 1980s some patients (e.g. young children) are best treated by traditional tube pedicle repair.

Tissue expansion before skin transfer, recently introduced, is also likely to improve results in burns contracture surgery in years to come.

Circumferential scars

Constricting scars around the whole circumference of a limb or the trunk are only seen if the original burn has been very deep, or primary repair has been long delayed or non-existent, by reason of lack of facilities or continued sepsis. Tightness which is sufficient to cause a contour defect should be released by longitudinal incision and free graft (*Figure 8.8*).

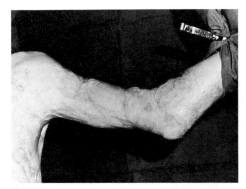

(a)

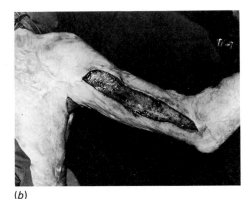

(b)

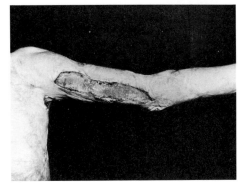

(c)

Figure 8.8 (*a*) Circumferential scar of the arm. This is the type of contracture which may lead to unstable scars and frank malignancy in the long term. (*b*) Simple full length incision leads to wide gaping of the wound. (*c*) Repair by free skin graft gives relief and long-term stability

Unstable scars

These scars are usually situated on extensor surfaces, and may be adherent to deep fascia, muscle or bone. They can also develop on a flexor surface after a very long interval in a tight circumferential scar. It is highly desirable to eliminate the unstable portion of the scar, to avoid the possible development of malignancy (Marjolin's ulcer, *Figure 8.9*). If the scar is unstable merely because it is too tight, relief of tightness by incision and free grafting will suffice; if it is adherent to bone or tendon, a pedicled repair is usually necessary.

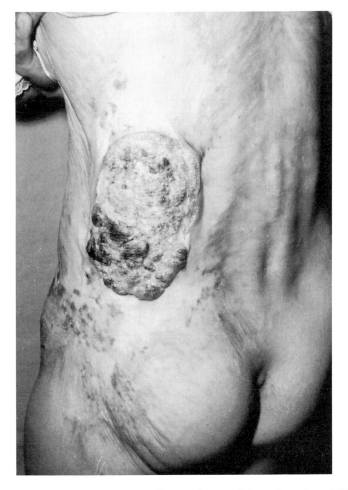

Figure 8.9 Frank epithelioma 67 years after sustaining a circumferential burn of the trunk

References

BARCLAY, T. L. (1986) Secondary surgery for burns. In *Operative Surgery Plastic Surgery,* 4th edn. London: Butterworths

HYNES, W. (1957) The treatment of scars by shaving and skin graft. *British Journal of Plastic Surgery,* **10,** 1

LARSON, D. L., ABSTON, A. S., EVANS, E. B., DOBRAKOWSKY, M., WILLIS, B. and LINARES, H. (1971) Development and correction of burns scar contracture. In *Research in Burns. Transactions of Third International Congress on Research in Burns.* Prague (1970). Bern: Hans Huber

MOWLEM, R. (1952) Hypertrophic scars. *British Journal of Plastic Surgery,* **4,** 113

Chapter 9

Administrative aspects of burns

Burns are common injuries, seen and treated by members of many different branches of the medical profession; they come within the ambits of general practitioners, casualty officers, general and orthopaedic surgeons engaged in traumatology, and plastic surgeons.

In the United Kingdom at the present time, patients with burns are usually seen first by the general practitioner or the casualty officer of the nearest hospital. If an ambulance is called to the site of the accident, the patient will be taken to the nearest hospital which has an accident department. Minor burns will continue to be treated by the general practitioner or casualty officer, while patients with more severe burns requiring in-patient hospital treatment will be admitted to the nearest general hospital, either under the care of the accident surgeon if he runs a comprehensive accident department, or under a general surgeon.

The disposal of the patient from then on depends on a number of factors. If the surgeon in the general hospital has an interest in treating burns and the nearest plastic surgery centre is difficult of access, some burns of intermediate size will remain under his care for definitive treatment. More commonly the surgeon's interests lie elsewhere and, if the patient can easily be transferred to the care of the plastic surgeon, this is what will usually be done. All serious burns will, either immediately or at an early stage, be transferred to a centre having special facilities for treatment of burns and, with a few special exceptions, this will be the regional plastic surgery centre.

The development of plastic surgery centres on a regional basis was due first to the demands of World War II and later to the organization of hospital services at the inception of the National Health Service in 1948. In the early part of the war, four main plastic surgery centres were established in the vicinity of London, and these were followed later by a small number of centres in other parts of England and Scotland. One of the main tasks of the plastic surgery services during the war was to deal with burning injuries in both servicemen and civilians. When the National Health Service was instituted, the existing services were taken over to provide plastic surgery services for the regional hospital board areas, and more centres were developed until each regional board area (with the exception of the northern region of Scotland) had its own centre. All these centres have facilities for treating extensive burns and in some, but not all, the patients are grouped together in a burns ward or burns unit. The burns unit at Birmingham Accident Hospital has developed along slightly different lines and holds a unique position in the country; not only is it the largest single unit, serving a densely populated and heavily industrialized area, but in addition has a close relationship with the Medical Research Council and has exceptional facilities for research.

In addition to the major regional plastic surgery centres mentioned above, a number of the large general hospitals now have plastic surgery units with facilities for the treatment of severe burns, giving a subregional service, and some of the larger children's hospitals also provide special accommodation for the treatment of burned children.

In the war-time plastic surgery centres, treatment of burns patients was in ordinary wards; after 1948 attempts were made to construct special accommodation in various centres so that the Burns Units at Birmingham, Roehampton, Mount Vernon and Glasgow were adaptations within existing wards, giving accommodation in single and shared rooms and providing an air-conditioned dressings room.

The first centre built specifically for burns treatment in the United Kingdom was that at Wakefield in 1964; this was followed by East Grinstead in 1965 and Salisbury in 1966. These units differ in many details but have all been built on similar lines, and designed to give maximum conventional protection against infection (within the limits of the money available). The newer units at Mount Vernon, Chepstow, Billericay and Aberdeen use modern air-engineering techniques to give increased protection against infection.

Knowledge gained from the work carried out in these units over the last two decades makes some observations possible, both on the future policy for the treatment of burns patients and on the design of their accommodation. Experience has shown that there are arguments both for and against the segregation of patients with burns into special units.

The arguments *in favour* are:

(1) These injuries require a high grade of expertise of medical and more particularly of nursing care, and this expertise can be achieved and maintained only by frequent practice.
(2) Patients with severe burns are at great risk particularly from infection, and need special facilities to minimize this risk. These facilities are expensive and need a high rate of usage if the expense is to be justified.

The arguments *against* are:

(1) The presence of large numbers of patients in close proximity very much increases the likelihood of cross-infection.

   During the 1950s and 1960s this was such a serious problem that, on occasion, burns units had to be closed completely because cross-infection had reached catastrophic proportions due to the large reservoir of infection that had built up. Now, thanks largely to the newer antiseptics, cross-infection and its deleterious effect is much less difficult to control.
(2) Burned patients make very heavy demands on nursing staff time and the staff requirements are much greater than in other surgical wards.

   Up to a certain size (in our view about 20 beds), these demands can be met within the overall nursing establishment of a major general hospital. When more patients than this have to be dealt with, there is a great danger, in view of conflicting demands and the ever-present nursing shortage, of the ward becoming understaffed, with consequent deterioration of standards.
(3) Patients with relatively small burns do not require special accommodation or elaborate facilities, and can be dealt with in ordinary surgical wards.

(4) If all burns facilities are centralized in special units and no provision is made for burns treatment in general hospitals, this will mean that many patients will be treated at considerable distance from their homes. This is a particularly important consideration in the case of children. Parents will gladly accept the inconvenience of having to make long trips to visit their child if they can understand that special facilities are vital for recovery, but if special measures are not necessary, they would much prefer treatment to be carried out at the nearest general hospital.

Three other considerations are relevant:

(1) The arrangements for the treatment of burns should integrate with the treatment of other injuries in the accident service.
(2) If the patient is to be treated in a general hospital, he should be admitted under the care of the plastic surgeon if one is available. No other surgeon is so well equipped by training and experience to deal with the problems of skin replacement and the more complicated methods of repair which may be necessary. In most of the accident services in the United Kingdom, the services of a plastic surgeon are readily available.
(3) Any burns unit or burns ward should be an integral part of the main plastic surgery centre. Experience in this country has shown that this arrangement has been markedly successful. It allows continuous 24-hour cover by experienced surgeons, it is desirable for training purposes and, even if only vicariously through juniors, it keeps the more senior plastic surgeon in touch with the burns problem.

The Accident Services Review Committee recommended in 1961 that the development of accident departments in district general hospitals (of approximately 800 beds) would provide a service for 100 000–200 000 people, and this has largely been achieved. The provision of highly specialized treatment for those who need it in a central accident unit located in a teaching hospital complex where specialities such as thoracic surgery, neurosurgery and plastic surgery would all be available, has not come to pass except in one or two regions; it seems unlikely that such a development in the hospital service will be forthcoming generally. If such a major reorganization does take place, the treatment of burns can fit in with the arrangements provided that the accident service at the district general hospital has facilities for:

(1) Resuscitation of major burns.
(2) Retention and definitive treatment of extensive superficial burns, and deep burns of up to 5 per cent surface area not involving either the hands or face.
(3) Out-patient treatment for minor burns.

Other than the normal facilities of an accident department, the unit would require only two single rooms, air conditioned to good modern standards (for shock treatment and assessment); the rooms would not need to be reserved exclusively for burns treatment, but could be used for other patients as well.

The burns ward connected with the regional accident service and with the regional plastic surgery centre could then adopt a selective policy and admit from the whole region all serious deep burns of the face and hands and burns with more than 5 per cent whole thickness skin loss; this would of course include all life-threatening injuries. We believe, however, that the burns centre should also admit and treat less serious cases from nearby. It is an error to plan for large and serious injuries only, and the functioning of the centre and the morale of its staff are much improved by having a steady proportion of less serious injuries, whose presence enables the routine to continue to function smoothly even when few serious injuries are admitted, and whose rapid and good recovery gives some relief from the strain of caring continuously for patients who are desperately ill for long periods, many of whom die. A unit of manageable size would consist of special accommodation for two to four badly burned patients and 8–16 beds for less serious injuries, and for the seriously injured patients when they have progressed beyond the need for special accommodation. The total number of beds would vary according to the size of the population served and the degree of selection, but a well balanced unit for a population of two million could be formed of four special rooms and 10 others. We do not consider that, except under special circumstances, any single unit should have a total of more than 20 beds.

Should the same unit care for both adults and children? There are arguments both for and against this view. If a comprehensive children's hospital is available, there are strong reasons for treating all children in an environment which is specially geared to their needs, but this is only true, certainly in the case of major burns, if the treatment given is of equal standard to that in a special department. On the other hand, it is certain that the morale of both medical and nursing staff in a burns unit is materially benefited by seeing badly injured children survive and prosper (*Figure 9.1*). This offsets some of the gloom and despondency engendered by the high mortality among the elderly. During the intensive care stage, when

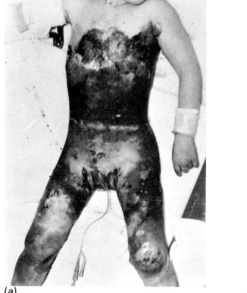

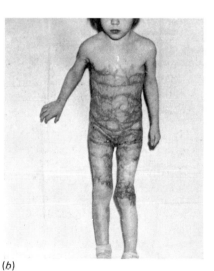

(a)   (b)

Figure 9.1 (*a*) Fifty-five per cent whole thickness burn from burning nightdress in a 4-year-old girl; the face and hands are uninvolved. (*b*) Eight weeks later; although more skin is required at the level of the groins, treatment of the potentially fatal injury has been well worthwhile. (Reprinted from T. L. Barclay, 1967, Management of burns, *Hospital Medicine*, pp. 1138–1149 with permission of the Publishers)

strict segregation is necessary, we have not encountered any serious objections to the mixing of ages in one unit. Although the highest incidence of burns is in the pre-school group, if a selective policy of treating mostly severe burns is followed, it will be found that a ward taking patients of all ages will admit approximately equal numbers of children and adults.

Design of burns units

A brief discussion of the principles of design of an orthodox burns unit, as at Wakefield, is appropriate here.

In the orthodox unit the accommodation is planned to take account of the two phases of the burns illness – the shock period and the healing period. Some patients will be admitted soon after the injury, at which time it is hoped that they will not be contaminated with pathogenic organisms, but they will be in danger from the development of shock. The essentials for the treatment of these acutely ill patients are plenty of space in which to work and cleanliness of the environment. The 'shock room' should, therefore, be as large as possible. Some form of air-conditioning is highly desirable. Adequate facilities for washing by the staff are essential, as is also a supply of oxygen and a suction apparatus. The patient will normally remain in this room for two or three days, at the end of which time he will no longer need transfusion. If treated by exposure, his burns will have dried or, alternatively, if treated by dressings, a definitive dressing will have been applied. He will then be ready for transfer to one of the ordinary rooms in the ward, which need not be as spacious as the shock room. An air-conditioned dressings room with a bath is essential; for operative procedures, an operating theatre in close proximity to the ward is highly desirable, although for considerations of expense it may not be possible to have an operating theatre reserved exclusively for burns patients.

The rooms themselves do not need to be as large as the shock room, but it may be necessary to use special cranes or beds and other apparatus for handling heavy patients, or those with coincidental other injuries; similarly such procedures as application of grafts while the patient is in his bed are often required, so that the room must be of adequate size. We believe that by far the best design of the patients' accommodation, for use after the shock phase is over, is two wings or corridors with duplicated services for each. A number of patients will be admitted with their burns already infected, and others will acquire infection in the burns centre, in particular by *Pseudomonas aeruginosa*. It is highly desirable that any patients whose burns are so colonized should be separated as far as possible from those who are not infected, by keeping the two groups of patients in separate wings, as it has not been found possible, even by strictly applied barrier nursing, to prevent cross-infection of patients in contiguous or nearby rooms. This design has an additional advantage that major maintenance, such as decorating and plastering, can be undertaken at less busy seasons without closing the burns unit completely.

Each wing of the ward block should contain several single rooms, each with separate toilet facilities. A proportion may be double rooms, but it seems unwise to plan for larger rooms than this; nor should more than half the beds be in shared rooms. Each room must have a television set as this has been found to be essential for preventing boredom and maintaining morale. Each wing requires a day room for patients who are ambulant and are considered suitable for mixing with others at a similar stage of their illness; unless, that is, a system of progressive patient care is in operation whereby, by the time the patient is ambulant, he is moved out into a separate ward.

A dressing station, which should include a bath with a mechanical hoist and a large area where major dressings can be done, is another vital part of the burns department. The bath and hoist are usually made of stainless steel which is easily cleaned and disinfected and there must be ample surfaces for the preparation of dressings. Air-conditioning to provide at least 12 and preferably 20 changes of air per hour is essential, as shown many years ago by Colebrook (1950). We believe that two complete dressing stations should be provided, if possible, one for each wing of the burns ward.

Finally, as in all departments, adequate storage space is essential; there are many items of bulky equipment in occasional use in burns wards, and great difficulties will be encountered if these have to be stored at a distance rather than being readily available.

The plan of the Burns Centre at Pinderfields Hospital is appended (*Figure 9.2*). This department has now been in continuous use for 20 years and has worked well in practice. It is depicted here not because we think it ideal, but because it may provide a starting point for other designs. It is not too elaborate. It would certainly

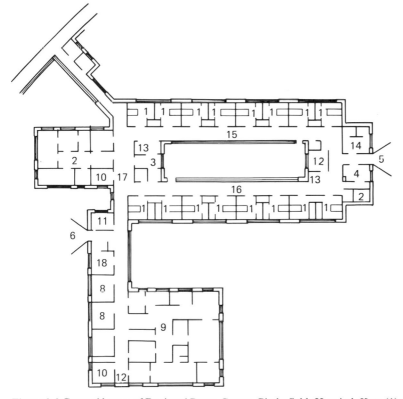

Figure 9.2 General layout of Regional Burns Centre, Pinderfields Hospital. Key: (1) single bedrooms; (2) dressings suite; (3) ward kitchen; (4) consultant's office; (5) visitors' entrance; (6) patients' entrance; (7) staff entrance; (8) resuscitation rooms; (9) theatre suite; (10) Sisters' office; (11) secretary's office; (12) sluices; (13) nurses' stations; (14) visitors' rooms; (15) north corridor; (16) south corridor; (17) main corridor; (18) patient reception

be improved by having a day room in each wing and by having two dressing stations instead of one. The patient rooms were not provided with air-conditioning because of cost considerations and it is still not certain how desirable it is to have this facility; air-conditioning is confined to the dressing room suite and the operating theatre suite. It was found shortly after the unit opened in 1965 that the original siting of the plant in the dressing room, by which the air was taken in from the exterior and exhausted into the main corridor of the ward accommodation, was causing gross contamination of the patients' accommodation in the 'clean' corridor; fortunately it was possible to rectify this so that air is now taken in from the corridor and exhausted to the outside. Each single room has a toilet and wash-handbasin *en suite*. Each patient's room, the shock room and the treatment rooms have disposal hatches which open by a baffle to the exterior, so that contaminated material can be collected outside without having to be transported through any other area. The cost of this department, including site preparation, construction and equipment was £123 000 at 1964 prices. The overall rate of infection for *Pseudomonas aeruginosa* has remained virtually stationary for the last 19 years, at about 30 per cent, so that avoidance of contamination of patient's wounds is very far from complete (Settle, 1985). It is probable that colonization by *Pseudomonas* is delayed by segregation of patients whose wounds are infected from those who are 'clean', and this in itself must be beneficial; first isolation of *Pseudomonas* now occurs on average on day 13, as opposed to day 16 in 1966–71, so that even such protection as this design of accommodation affords is gradually declining after nearly two decades of continuous use.

Air-conditioning has now become an accepted feature of new hospital building and is used, not only to give improved conditions of comfort, but also to provide a bacteriologically clean atmosphere and thus diminish the risk of cross-infection in the hospital wards. It should be remembered, however, that conventional air-conditioning acts in the latter context by a continuous dilution effect and the ambient air still contains a small population of bacteria. Because of the natural defence mechanisms of the body, these sparse bacteria do little harm to the ordinary surgical patient but the burned patient is in different circumstances. Not only does he have a large open wound which is present in the operating theatre during the course of a surgical operation, but also his natural defence mechanism may be severely depressed by his injury. The atmosphere in the room of the severely burned patient should therefore be at least as clean as the air in a modern operating theatre and, indeed, there are good grounds for suggesting that it should be as clean as the operating enclosures which the orthopaedic surgeons use for the operations of inserting artificial joints.

For the immediate future, therefore, any new burns facility should have the patients' rooms ventilated to a high standard of cleanliness (i.e. to present operating theatre standards) and a dressings room with air-conditioning of similar quality. In addition, the whole department should have an overall balanced system of pressures which will ensure that no air flows from contaminated to clean areas or to other patients.

It should, however, be remembered that, although positive pressure air-conditioning does afford valuable extra protection for the high risk patient, it may have been dearly bought if accompanied by cramping of the accommodation, since in the event of mechanical breakdown heavy cross-infection would then be certain.

The new unit in Aberdeen uses more advanced air engineering techniques which have been pioneered in the orthopaedic operation field. More operational studies need to be carried out to know if this approach will prove to be sufficiently effectively to justify its cost.

Mass casualties

Mass casualties involving a large number of patients with burns injuries require special consideration. It behoves all health authorities and clinicians running accident departments to be prepared, in so far as is reasonable, by prior planning, to cope with the casualties from a burns catastrophe.

During the last 25 years several burns incidents have been sufficiently documented for a number of common factors both in the type of injury and in the best disposal of the patients to be identified. The circus fire at Niteroi in Brazil in 1961 (Pitanguy, 1965), when 400 patients died in or shortly after the conflagration (and many of the patients who reached hospital alive succumbed later), the Circus Fire at Bangalore in 1981 (Das, 1983), with 77 immediate and 24 subsequent fatalities, and the camping ground expolosion at Los Alfaques in 1978 (Arthurson, 1981) in which 102 people perished immediately and 108 later, all resulted in serious burns on a massive scale, but the treatment available immediately and also later on differed considerably. Catastrophies in this country have been on a smaller scale, which include the Summerland Leisure Complex fire in 1973 and the Bradford Football Stand fire in 1985 (Sharpe et al., 1985; Barclay, 1986), and the number of patients with severe burns who reached hospital were fewer in number. In every one of these incidents the burns casualties have been of six main types:

(1) Dead.
(2) Inevitably fatal.
(3) Life-threatening by reason of extent of burn.
(4) Life-threatening by reason of inhalation injury.
(5) Disabling but not life-threatening.
(6) Minor burns treatable as out-patients.

Because the facilities necessary for optimum treatment of each type of injury vary so greatly, expert initial sorting is of paramount importance.

The dead
Although the hospital is not involved, a vast amount of work remains for police and rescue services in identification and disposal of fatal casualties.

The patients with injuries which by reason of age and extent of burn will inevitably be fatal (see Chapter 1)
The specialist burns department normally accepts patients in this category in single numbers from individual domestic and industrial accidents, despite the known outcome. When the department's special facilities are at a premium, to deal with life-threatening, but not inevitably fatal, burns in large numbers, no room will be available for the patients who, experience shows, will inevitably die of their injuries within the next few days. It would be totally wrong and inhumane to admit these patients and then transfer them elsewhere to die in order to accommodate potential survivors; the fatally injured must never be sent to the special department in these desperate circumstances. They should be admitted either to the intensive care wards of surrounding hospitals if enough accommodation exists, or to a special ward requisitioned *ad hoc*, depending on the numbers involved.

Life-threatening major body burns

These are the patients who must have first class treatment in special accommodation if they are to have the best chance of survival. A specialist burns centre is very unlikely to be able to admit more than six of these patients at once, if that; disperal to other burns departments on a regional or national basis would have to be arranged if the numbers exceed six. If patients in this category were numbered in hundreds, some with only the slimmest chance of survival might have to be relegated to the previous category, so that the actual extent of burn which can be judged fatal might in exceptional circumstances have to be varied.

Inhalation injury

The best place for these patients is the intensive care ward, under the supervision not of burns surgeons but of anaesthetists and chest physicians. The need for intubation and tracheostomy is a very special problem (*see* Chapter 5). A patient who has surface burns and a significant inhalation injury has a markedly worse prognosis than a patient with comparable surface burns alone; a method of clinical scoring combined with carboxyhaemoglobin estimation has been elaborated by Clark and his colleagues (1986) to assess the increased mortality probability.

Disabling burns which require hospital treatment but which are not likely to be life-threatening

Burns of up to 20 per cent of the body surface are, except in elderly patients, in this category, and in the mass casualty situation there will not be room for these patients in the specialist burns centre. Prior planning should therefore identify accommodation at the local general hospital which can be made available at short notice for reception and treatment of these patients, whose hospital stay can be

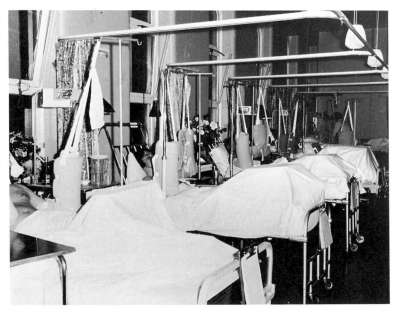

Figure 9.3 Large number of intravenous drip stands in use when 63 patients with burns of the hands were admitted to hospital after the Bradford Football Stand Fire (1985)

expected to extend to a few weeks. Extra staff, both surgical and nursing, with a good knowledge of burns care may have to be recruited.

Patients who can, at any rate to begin with, be treated as out-patients
The numbers will again depend on the size of the disaster – in a very great catastrophe hospital accommodation might simply not be available for anyone who could possibly walk or care for themselves, but even for manageable civilian disasters the number of out-patients may be very large and provide a considerable load for the hospital; 148 such patients were treated on an out-patient regime following the Bradford fire. A special clinic will have to be organized for these patients, and knowledgeable staff provided.

Criteria for assessing the need for intravenous resuscitation may also vary in extreme circumstances, but usually shock will not be manifest in children with burns of less than 10 per cent of the body surface, or 15 per cent in adults (*Figure 9.3*). It is perhaps better to erect an intravenous infusion and subsequently to discontinue it if reassessment makes it clear that it is unnecessary than to postpone such a task until the patient is very ill and all his veins in spasm. Large numbers of infusion sets and drip stands will be required in any event, and planners must be aware of this vital need.

In summary, prior planning should be directed to identifying experienced doctors who can accurately assess the casualties when they are first seen, to earmarking accommodation in the local hospital for patients with non-life-threatening injuries, to making sure that lines of communication with the regional burns centre and the intensive care wards of surrounding hospitals are easily opened, and to considering how a very large number of outpatient burns can best be cared for in the accommodation available (*see Figure 9.4*).

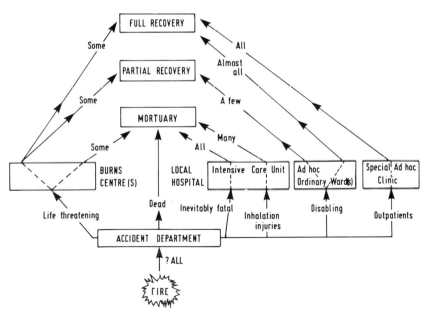

Figure 9.4 Flow-chart for patients burned in a major catastrophe

References

ARTURSON, G. (1981) The Los Alfaques Disaster: a boiling liquid expanding vapour explosion. *Burns,* **7,** 233–251

BARCLAY, T. L. (1986) Planning for mass burns casualties. Royal Society of Medicine Services. *Round Table Series No. 3.* Ed. C. Wood. *Accident and Emergency Burns Lessons from the Bradford Disaster*

CLARK, C. J., REID, W. H., GILMORE, W. H. and CAMPBELL, D. (1986) Mortality probability of victims of fire trauma: revised equation to include inhalation injury. *British Medical Journal,* **292,** 1303–1305

COLEBROOK, L. (1950) *A New Approach to Treatment of Burns and Scalds.* London: Fine Technical Publications

DAS, R. A. P. (1983) Circus fire at Bangalore. *Burns,* **10,** 17–29

PITANGUY, I. (1965) Treatment of victims of the great catastrophe in the Gran circus at Niteroi. In *Research in Burns. Transactions of the Second International Congress on Research in Burns,* p. 216. Edinburgh: E & S Livingstone

SETTLE, J. A. D. (1985) Infection in burns. *Journal of Hospital Infection,* **6,** Suppl. B

SHARPE, D. T., ROBERTS, A. H. N., BARCLAY, T. L., DICKSON, W. A., SETTLE, J. A. D., CROCKETT, D. J. *et al.* (1985) Treatment of burns casualties after fire at Bradford City Football Club Ground. *British Medical Journal,* **291,** 945–949

Further reading

BARCLAY, T. L. (1967) Control of *Ps. pyocyanea* in the Regional Burns Centre, Wakefield. *Journal of Royal College of Surgeons of Edinburgh,* **12,** 250

BARCLAY, T. L. (1970) *Pseudomonas aeruginosa* in relation to burns. *ChM Thesis.* University of Edinburgh

BARCLAY, T. L. and DEXTER, F. (1968) Infection and cross-infection in a new burns centre. *British Journal of Surgery,* **55,** 197

BEECH, W. (1955) Burns casualties from H.M.S. *Indomitable. British Journal of Plastic Surgery,* **7,** 303

OSMOND-CLARKE, H. (1961) *Report of Accident Services Review Committee.* London: British Medical Association

Index